Aromatherapy for Self-Care

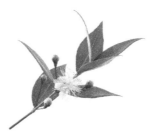

Aromatherapy

FOR SELF-CARE

**Your Complete Guide *to* Relax, Rebalance,
and Restore *with* Essential Oils**

SARAH SWANBERG, MS, LAC

PHOTOGRAPHY © ANNIE MARTIN

ROCKRIDGE
PRESS

Interior and Cover Designer: Tricia Jang

Editor: Rachel Feldman

Production Editor: Emily Sheehan

Photography: © 2019 Annie Martin. Styling by Jenna Baucke

ISBN: Print 978-1-64611-221-0 | eBook 978-1-64611-222-7

R0

For my Brownies,
I love you to the sky and back.

CONTENTS

INTRODUCTION

Welcome to the world of aromatherapy! Since you are reading this, I am guessing you are interested in practicing more self-care in your life—and you are in luck, because using essential oils is a great way to start. Aromatherapy, or the therapeutic use of essential oils, has been gaining in popularity—and it is no surprise why. Our fast-paced, overly processed world has made it more important than ever to find natural ways to de-stress. Plus, all you need to get started are essential oils, a nose, and a set of lungs (and I am willing to bet you already have some of those things).

As an acupuncturist, I often use essential oils while treating patients. I find lavender incredibly helpful in getting patients relaxed for an acupuncture treatment and citrus oil blends are great for reenergizing them after a blissful "acu-nap." At home, I use essential oils with my kids, for cleaning products, and for my own self-care practices. Before you start assuming that I am an all-natural, crunchy, no-store-bought-anything hippie mama, let me also tell you that I do keep stronger, store-bought cleaning products and over-the-counter medicines in my home, too. I am all about practicality and I believe there is a time and a place for everything. But going natural is always my first resort, and to be honest, I very rarely have to break out the synthetic stuff.

I am so grateful for the lifesaving medications that our pharmaceutical industry provides, which often enable people to live longer, fuller lives, but stronger medications often come with bigger side effects and they are not always necessary. Tapping into the healing powers of the natural world around us and within our own bodies is immensely powerful. It is something I work with and witness on a daily basis. Our bodies truly do have an incredible capacity to heal. Learning to trust that ability takes time, but I am happy you are on your way. Let me be the first to welcome you to the club!

My goal with this book is to help you use aromatherapy to improve your emotional, mental, and physical well-being—naturally. We will dive into the importance of self-care, the role aromatherapy can play, and what tools you will need to make it happen. I will also provide you with 100 remedies for emotional, mental, and physical self-care.

I am so excited to introduce you to this powerful (and wonderfully fragrant) world as you take this amazing step on your self-care journey!

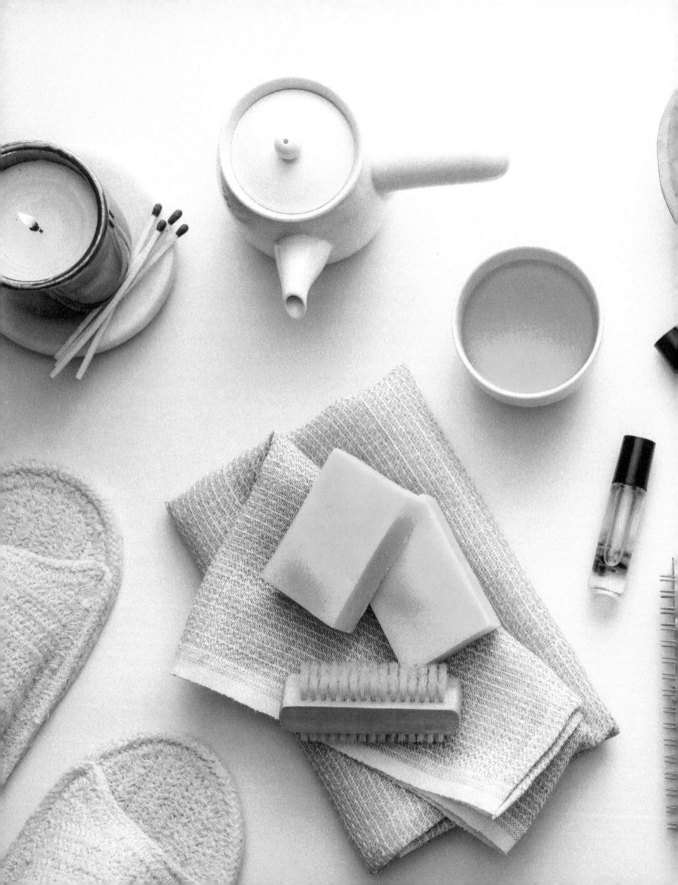

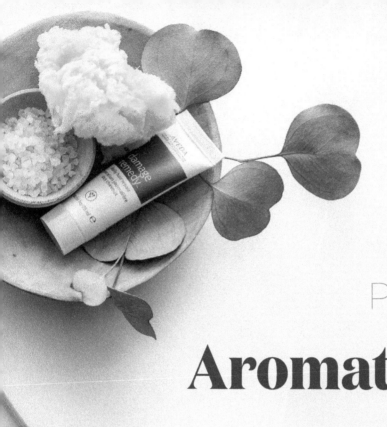

PART ONE

Aromatherapy *for the* Real World

This part starts with a bird's-eye view of self-care and aromatherapy. You will learn how aromatherapy can help improve your overall well-being and also help you target specific issues. You will also get familiar with each of the essential oils that are used in the remedies in part 2 and figure out which tools you need to get started. Consider this your Aromatherapy 101 course!

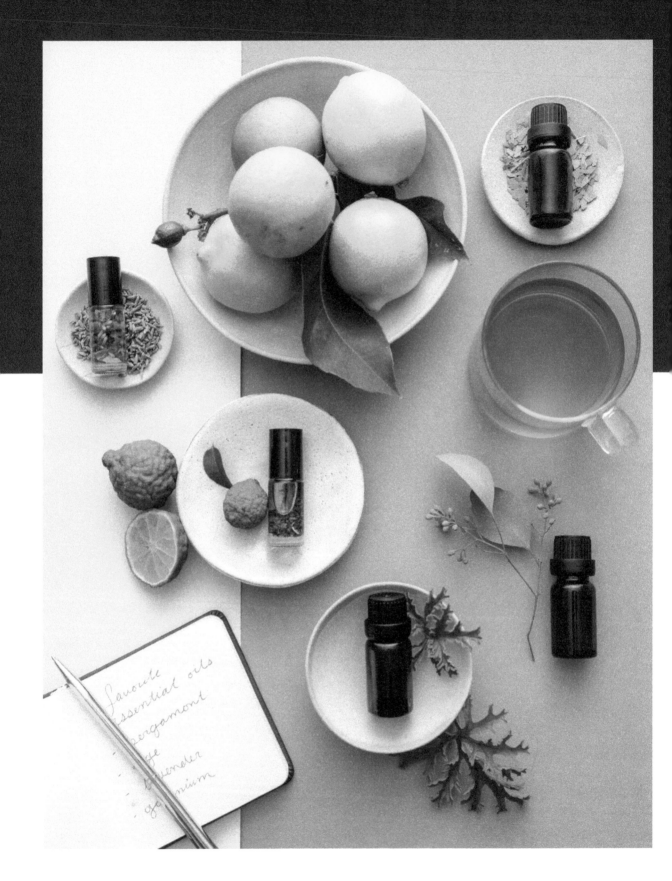

Self-Care and Aromatherapy

Before we dive into aromatherapy and its potential benefits for your overall health and wellness, we first need to discuss what self-care is and why it is important. This chapter covers why you should care about self-care, how it can impact your life, and why it is important to use self-care to help prevent issues rather than just treat them. Picking up a book like this is a great form of self-care, so hooray, you are already a step ahead of the game! Now let's take a few deep breaths (yep, that is a self-care practice), get yourself a glass of water or tea (self-care, too!), and let's dig in.

CARING ABOUT SELF-CARE

If you have spent any time on the Internet in the last decade, you have probably seen the term "self-care" thrown about. You may have seen it applied to ultra-luxe spa visits or to simple discussions on basic nutrients—and everything in between. Before we take a look at how different people define "self-care," first we need to talk about why self-care is such a hot topic.

Life is a bit more complicated these days than it used to be. You may find yourself juggling many things at once—career, education, family, and hobbies—and the effort it takes to balance it all can easily start to affect your health and well-being. Stress has become a major issue in our lives. We are always on the go to keep up with demanding jobs, active social lives, bills to pay, errands to run, families and friends to care for, and social media to endlessly browse! I am partly joking about that last one, but modern technology does play a big role in our daily stress. Many of us have a hard time disconnecting from our devices, which leads to difficulty disconnecting in general. This combination of being overworked and overstimulated has created a need for more conscious self-care practices to help balance our busy lives and keep us grounded and healthy. Self-care is very important to keep this juggle from turning into a struggle.

So, What Is Self-Care?

If you look the term up on the Internet, you will find a lot of different answers. Some people think of self-care as pampering. Though a day at the spa or a luxurious bath-time ritual can absolutely be beneficial, self-care is much more than the "treat yourself" variety popularized on Instagram. Other people define *self-care* as something you do to care for your own health and wellness, outside of the care that is provided by someone like a doctor, therapist, or counselor. According to this view, self-care would include paying your bills, brushing your teeth, hitting the gym, eating your veggies, booking that acupuncture appointment, and so on. It would also include saying no to things like one more pour of rosé wine or an extra project that you just do not have the bandwidth for.

I like to think of self-care as anything that helps you refill your gas tank. Close your eyes and imagine yourself as a car (I would be a vintage Aston Martin convertible, thank you very much). If you were driving around all day to and from meetings, school pickups, and family gatherings, you would need to have enough gas to get around. If the level got dangerously low, your fuel light would go off, reminding you to refill the tank. Our bodies work pretty similarly—we need physical, mental, and emotional fuel to perform all the tasks that our modern world asks of us. We do have low-fuel warnings—it just takes a little awareness to figure out what they are so that we do not end up running out of gas.

Recognizing those signals is only half the battle, though. The other half is regularly topping off your gas tank to keep that light from turning on in the first place. Self-care is taking an active and deliberate role in protecting your physical, mental, and emotional well-being, especially during stressful or challenging times.

Wondering where to start? The foundations of self-care include basic needs like sleep, exercise, and nutrition. These are vital to your overall wellness and should always be your first priority. After that, we have work, relationships, time with loved ones, and hobbies. Nourishing these aspects of your life helps prevent stress and burnout. At the top of the pyramid, you'll find all of the "extras"—things that we can add to our lives to reduce the stress burden and keep our tanks topped off. These include things like meditation, bodywork, time in nature, pampering, supplements, laughter, and—of course—aromatherapy!

SELF-CARE PYRAMID

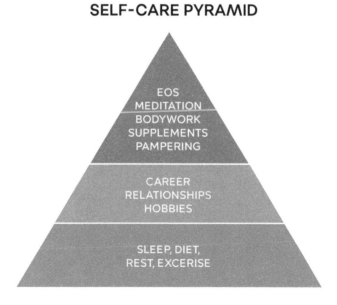

EOS
MEDITATION
BODYWORK
SUPPLEMENTS
PAMPERING

CAREER
RELATIONSHIPS
HOBBIES

SLEEP, DIET,
REST, EXCERISE

A moment of real talk: If you care for other people, whether personally or professionally, you might find the idea of self-care slightly selfish. How could you, you might wonder, take time for yourself when your priority is supporting others? Well, just remember what they tell you in those airplane safety demonstrations: You have to put on your own oxygen mask before helping others put on theirs. If you are not getting oxygen yourself, you are pretty much no help to anyone else.

Mini-Guides for Self-Care

Part 2 of this book offers 100 remedies for taking care of your emotional, mental, and physical wellness, but if you want to get your feet wet right away, here are some mini-guides to help you get started.

Morning Boost

Maybe you didn't get solid sleep thanks to a late-night Netflix binge, or maybe you just could not stop thinking about *everything*. Whatever the reason, if you wake up feeling groggy, this mini-guide is for you. Try a remedy like the **QUICK PICK-ME-UP INHALER** (see page 124) or grab an uplifting essential oil like eucalyptus or grapefruit and use one of the following methods:

DIFFUSER. Right after you wake up, add a few drops of the remedy blend or essential oil to your essential oil diffuser. As it gets going, take a few moments to stretch or practice mindful breathing for some extra self-care gold stars. Once the oil is being diffused into the air, continue mindful breathing as you get ready to start your day.

SHOWER. Don't have time to diffuse? Add a drop or two of the oil to a washcloth and place it on your shower floor. My personal favorite is eucalyptus to get that at-home spa vibe. For an added bonus, inhaling the fragrant steam can also help clear sinus congestion.

ON THE GO. Don't forget that the easiest method of aromatherapy is just a simple, deep inhalation. Keeping a bottle of essential oil in your bag or at your desk and just taking a good whiff can be enough to give you a quick boost. (If you are a car commuter, place a drop of essential oil on a cotton ball and stick it between the slats of your air vent as a quickie diffuser. I love to do this with citrus blends. It wakes me up and keeps my car smelling great!)

Calm Mind

Anxious about a work meeting or an upcoming date (go, you!), or just feeling overwhelmed? First, find a calm, quiet place where you can take some slow, deep breaths to help your body settle down. Square breathing—breathing in to a count of four, holding for a count of four, breathing out for a count of four, and holding for a count of four—is a really quick way to settle your nervous system. Pick a remedy like the **ANTIANXIETY INHALER** (see page 79) or choose a calming essential oil like frankincense or geranium and use one of the following methods:

ROLLERBALL. A rollerball bottle is a small cylindrical bottle that makes applying prediluted essential oils quick and easy. All you need to do is uncap the bottle and roll the ball applicator along your skin to get the benefits. You can apply a rollerball to the inside of your wrists, along your collarbone, or on the back of your neck. You can even roll a bit into the palms of your hands and take some deep breaths while lifting your hands to your face.

JEWELRY DIFFUSER. Lava bead jewelry, made of porous lava stone, is another way to diffuse on the go—the porous stone absorbs the oil and allows you to keep smelling it all day long.

SELF-APPLICATION. Keep a diluted lavender essential oil in your desk drawer or bag and apply a drop of oil directly to acupressure points that have a calming and grounding effect, such as Pericardium 6 (located on the inner wrist) or Kidney 1 (located on the sole of the foot). (You can see an illustration of these points on page 37.)

Better Sleep

You probably already know that the amount of sleep you get is super important to your overall well-being, but the quality of sleep matters, too. Deep, restful sleep is when your body does most of its healing, and long-term sleep issues can have some pretty big ramifications. Try ending your exposure to all device screens at least one hour before bed, making sure your bedroom is dark and quiet (white-noise machines can help drown out unwanted noises), and lowering the temperature in your room, if possible. You can try doing a quick yoga pose, like legs-up-the-wall, before getting into bed. Then get some clary sage or lavender, which are two of the best essential oils for sleep, and try one of the following methods:

DIFFUSER. Turn your diffuser on before you get ready for bed, so by the time you tuck yourself under the covers, it is fully going. Creating a daily bedtime ritual can really help send a signal to your brain that it is time to turn off. I like to lower the lights, put on some peaceful music, and diffuse a few drops of lavender and Roman chamomile essential oils while I put on my pajamas. By the time I slide into bed, I am very relaxed and ready to head off to dreamland. If you tend to wake up in the middle of the night, try to use a diffuser that has a longer run-time setting to keep the diffusion going longer.

BATH. If a warm bath at night is in the cards, this is a *great* way to unwind. Adding Epsom salts (made with magnesium, which is naturally calming) combined with a few drops of a calming essential oil can really help release pent-up stress from the day and get you one step closer to a night full of z's. (And always combine essential oils with salt or a carrier oil before adding them to a bath to avoid skin sensitivity; you will learn more about this later.)

QUICK FIX. Don't have time for a lengthy bedtime ritual? Try applying a calming essential oil that has been properly diluted to the bottom of your feet, wrists, temples, or behind your ears. You can also try the **DREAMTIME PILLOW SPRAY** (see page 140).

YOUR OVERALL WELL-BEING

Remember that car analogy from earlier in this chapter? We are going to toss that one out of the passenger-side window now because your body is, in fact, nothing like a car. When a car part is broken, you can usually just replace that part and your car is as good as new. But our bodies do not work like this. Each part and every organ affects the whole system. We operate much more like a garden than a car—and for that garden to flourish, we need good soil, plenty of water, and sunlight. Think of each of these as our emotional, mental, and physical components that work together to create overall well-being.

In Western medicine, specialization (that is, physicians choosing just one area of medicine to study) has led to the compartmentalization of our health. But, in reality, every aspect of our health is connected. It is rare to find someone who feels emotionally fabulous but is physically unwell. Our physical, mental, and emotional health are very strongly linked—just think about how stress can cause headaches or digestive issues, depression can cause insomnia, and physical exhaustion can cause brain fog and lack of productivity. This is why it is important to look at the body as a whole when we think about self-care.

Emotional

Contrary to popular belief, emotional well-being does not mean feeling happy 24-7. It is about experiencing an appropriate balance of feelings and not getting stuck in patterns of emotions like anger, fear, or sadness. (Yes, you can even get stuck in joy; mental health professionals call that "mania.") Anger is sometimes completely appropriate. If someone cuts you off in traffic or steals your wallet, of course you should be mad. If a loved one passes away, grief is a normal and appropriate response. But if we lose our ability to move between emotions, we get stuck and that can cause repercussions in our mental and physical well-being. Emotional self-care includes activities like journaling, breath work, meditation, and therapy.

Mental

Mental and emotional well-being have a lot of overlap, but in this sense, I am talking about cognitive functions like memory, critical thinking, and the ability to concentrate. While short periods of stress can actually stimulate your brain and improve focus and concentration (think of all those deadline-induced all-nighters in college), chronic stress can eventually lead to brain fog and short-term memory issues. Mental self-care includes prioritizing sleep, taking "brain breaks" during periods of study or concentration, supplementing with nutrients like omega-3 fatty acids for cognition, and building your mental muscles with activities like crossword puzzles and sudoku.

Physical

Physical well-being is not just the absence of disease (but yes, that is important, too), but it also includes feeling energized, having the ability to fall asleep and stay asleep, experiencing no or little pain, and generally feeling good. We tend to be a little more aware of our physical well-being than anything else, but when we experience poor physical, mental, *and* emotional health, it can be hard to unravel whether the physical symptoms are the cause of or a result of the other issues. Physical self-care includes eating well, exercising regularly, and prioritizing sleep.

THE ROLE OF AROMATHERAPY

So, what exactly is aromatherapy and what does it have to do with self-care? Essential oils are powerful plant extracts, and their therapeutic use has proven benefits for physical, mental, and emotional well-being. The best part is that essential oils are completely natural, which makes them an especially great self-care tool in today's world where harmful synthetic chemicals are rampant.

Aromatherapy is not a magical cure-all, but it can have amazingly beneficial effects on your overall health and well-being. My goal with this book is to introduce you to ways to use essential oils to improve your self-care game, help you find relief from symptoms, and cope with the stresses of everyday life.

"Natural" Medicine?

Let's chat about the word "natural" for a second. This seemingly simple word carries *a lot* of baggage in today's world. Some opponents of natural health-care practices, especially herbal or plant medicines, argue that natural remedies are a waste of money. Often, they attribute any benefits to the placebo effect (where a treatment works only because the person using it believes it works). Others argue that natural remedies are potentially harmful and should be avoided. And then there are some who make outlandish, irresponsible, and downright dangerous claims about what natural remedies like essential oils can cure.

Aside from needing sunlight and water, plants are pretty self-sufficient, so it is no surprise that they can have potent effects on our health. That being said, just because something is natural does not mean that it is automatically safe—and it definitely does not mean that it is going to be a magical cure-all. Really, too much of anything, even something natural, can be bad for your health. But when compared with the safety of pharmaceuticals, which often contain powerful synthetic versions of plant ingredients, natural medicine has a pretty good safety record when used responsibly.

Because of a lack of regulation in the natural medicine world, you need to do your homework. This book is a step in the right direction. And of course, always discuss the use of essential oils and aromatherapy with your health-care practitioner, and do not use these remedies to replace things like necessary medication and therapy.

How It Works

You might be wondering exactly how a lovely smelling essential oil can help you reduce stress, lull you to sleep, and provide all the other health benefits mentioned in this book. Well, aromatherapy is believed to work by stimulating smell receptors in the nose, which then send messages through the nervous system to the limbic system (the part of your brain that controls memory and emotions). In addition to your nose, essential oil molecules can also enter through your skin when the oil is applied topically.

Let's take a look at how both of these methods work:

WHEN INHALED

Most of us do not spend too much time thinking about our sense of smell unless it activates our salivary glands, thanks to a delicious home-cooked meal, or if it sends a warning signal to our brain to alert us of a gas leak, fire, or spoiled food. But our sense of smell is way more important and a whole lot more complicated than that. Because scent signals interact with the body's nervous system and travel through its limbic system, that makes aromatherapy an amazing and powerful tool for affecting mood and overall well-being.

Because the molecules that make up essential oils are so tiny, they cross the blood-brain barrier, which is a layer of cells that keeps the brain safe from pathogens and other toxins (a feat most drugs and even some herbs are unable to accomplish). This means that the oils we smell are actually entering our brains, which makes these tiny molecules super powerful. Inhaling essential oils is the fastest and most effective method of aromatherapy. Consider this the express lane to your brain!

In case you were curious, this has all been backed up by science: The first officially published research on this topic came out in 1923, well before the invention of many of our modern-day medicines. It showed that smell has a direct effect on the central nervous system, including respiration and blood pressure. More recent studies have shown that smells have instant psychological *and* physiological effects, influencing feelings like attraction and repulsion.

This is where things can get tricky, though: Our sense of smell and our memory are closely connected. It is possible for a scent that is considered calming for most people to trigger a completely opposite emotion for someone else, based on their memories. For example, lavender calms most people, but if you had a nasty aunt who always wore lavender perfume, it could easily trigger feelings of hurt or anger. Keep these emotional connections in mind when searching for essential oils and blends that work for you.

WHEN APPLIED TOPICALLY

The topical application of essential oils has its merits, too. This method tends to work a bit more slowly and its effectiveness also depends on skin thickness and the extent of dilution, which is *always* recommended to prevent side effects (see the dilution chart on page 42).

Topical application can provide immediate benefits for skin issues, like stopping the itch from a mosquito bite, soothing the pain from a sunburn, or taking some of the sting out of a minor wound. It can also be used in the form of a chest rub to soothe coughs and congestion, a massage oil for muscle pains, and a soothing salve to relieve menstrual cramps, skin conditions, and acute muscle issues. And some acupuncturists (me included) use essential oils to stimulate certain acupuncture points in place of actual needles.

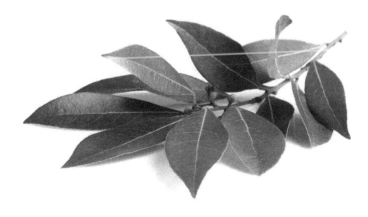

YOUR SELF-CARE PLAN

Now that you have all this information, what do you do with it? You might have one specific issue, like chronic back pain, for which you would like to use aromatherapy or you might have a bunch of issues going on and plan to be all-in with essential oils to support your overall well-being. To figure out how aromatherapy can work best for you, you will first need to determine your needs.

Enhancing Wellness Practices

Want to get the most bang for your buck when it comes to wellness practices like yoga or meditation? Add aromatherapy! Because aromatherapy is a passive practice (meaning you do not have to do much except breathe—which you should be doing about 15 times per minute anyway), you can easily combine it with other wellness practices to double the benefits.

You will often find aromatherapy as an add-on for services like massage, reflexology, and acupuncture—I personally love to include essential oils during my patients' acupuncture sessions for some extra R & R. You can "add-on" at home, too: Try using essential oils before turning on your favorite meditation app or diffuse a blend before rolling out a yoga mat to create a yoga studio vibe in your bedroom.

Determining Your Needs

This book focuses primarily on incorporating aromatherapy into your self-care practice, but before we get there, the first order of business is to do a little self-reflection to see what areas of your life are helping you fill that gas tank and which ones might be emptying it too fast. (You probably realize by now how much I love using this analogy. It just makes self-care so much easier to understand!)

Are you happy and fulfilled with your job? If not, start thinking about your career goals and make a plan for how to get there. Do you have satisfying relationships with people who make you feel good about yourself and support you? If not, it might be time to reevaluate those friendships. Are you eating a healthy diet? Food should be fun and enjoyable, but it can also really tip the scale toward health or toward illness (not to mention the huge impact that food choices have on our mood), so if there is room for improvement here, that is another great place to focus.

Since you picked up this book, I am guessing you already have a running list of things you would like to work on. But how exactly do you decide what to tackle first? As a Chinese medicine practitioner, I am trained to always look for the root cause of specific symptoms. I am going to teach you how to be your own root-cause detective here, which will then help you prioritize your needs and begin to devise a plan. When you look at your health through this lens, you might be surprised at what turns up.

Start by writing down a list of your symptoms. For example, your list might include the following:

- Anxiety
- Insomnia/trouble staying asleep
- Fatigue
- Sugar cravings in the afternoon

Now, let's take that list and see if we can find connections between any of the symptoms. Sugar cravings are likely due to fatigue, especially if they coincide with an afternoon energy slump. That fatigue is very likely due to difficulty sleeping. Anxiety can be both the cause of and a result of poor sleep, but in this case, let us assume that anxiety is *not* the cause here but just a symptom experienced after sleepless nights. Use arrows to point certain symptoms back to others, and then circle the symptom or symptoms that have the most arrows. This is most likely the root issue.

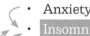

- Anxiety
- Insomnia/trouble staying asleep
- Fatigue
- Sugar cravings in the afternoon

Using this method helps us determine a plan. In this example, we want to focus on the sleep issues because solving that might actually relieve everything else on the list. If we treat the fatigue by using essential oils that are stimulating and energizing, that does not really get to the root of the problem and it might even make the sleep problems worse. If you are still unsure about where to focus, go back to the self-care pyramid (see page 3) and prioritize the issues at the base of the pyramid first.

What If It's Not Working for Me?

In today's next-day-delivery world, we are used to quick fixes and instant results. Remember that aromatherapy is not a magic bullet, and it might take some time to start noticing results. If you are frustrated and feeling like nothing is working, try some of these tips:

CHECK IN WITH YOURSELF. Maybe you have been using essential oils to help you feel more productive during the day, but if you have not been sleeping enough at night, there is only so much essential oils can do. Adding a nighttime routine with soothing essential oils might help you sleep better, eliminating the need for that daytime boost. Revisit your self-care plan to see if there is a potential root cause you are not considering. Also remember that the part of the brain that registers scent is closely related to the part that holds memories. Check in with yourself to see if an essential oil you are using might be triggering negative emotions because it brings up a bad memory. If so, use a different scent.

KEEP A JOURNAL. Sometimes it is difficult to notice subtle improvements. Keeping a journal can be incredibly helpful to show the bigger picture. For example, if you suffer from frequent headaches, jot down a note every time you get one. If you go from seven to five headaches a week, it may still feel like a lot of headaches, but you are actually improving. Keeping a detailed record like this over time can help you see even the littlest bits of progress, which often helps keep you motivated.

CHANGE IT UP. Regularly alternating essential oils is a good idea. It is possible to build up a tolerance to the effects of certain essential oils, and using a strong remedy in the same area for several days or weeks can cause skin irritation. The beauty of essential oils is that many different oils have similar properties. If you feel like one of them is not working or you are not seeing the same effects that you used to have, switch it up. If, for example, you diffuse lavender at bedtime but you still do not feel sleepy, try another relaxing oil instead, such as clary sage.

Making a Plan

So now that you have a goal (peaceful, restful z's), it is time to come up with the game plan. Go through part 2 of this book to find the blends that fit your root symptom(s) and which essential oils they use. With essential oils, always start slowly to make sure you do not experience any adverse effects. It is super-important to note that if you *do not* like the scent of a certain oil, skip it. One of the reasons that aromatherapy is so effective is that it can quickly affect our moods, so if a scent makes you cringe, it is not going to help!

Depending on your specific needs and goals, you might want to use aromatherapy as a treatment when symptoms arise (as with headaches) or as a prevention to avoid symptoms (like before a big meeting where you might typically experience anxiety). Keep track of the results by using a journal or a notes app on your smartphone. Pay attention to a decrease in the severity or frequency of your symptoms. Also, jot down if you had better results diffusing oils or using them topically. Yes, there is a science to using essential oils, but a lot of this comes down to your own personal experience, which often takes some experimentation. So be a good scientist and take notes!

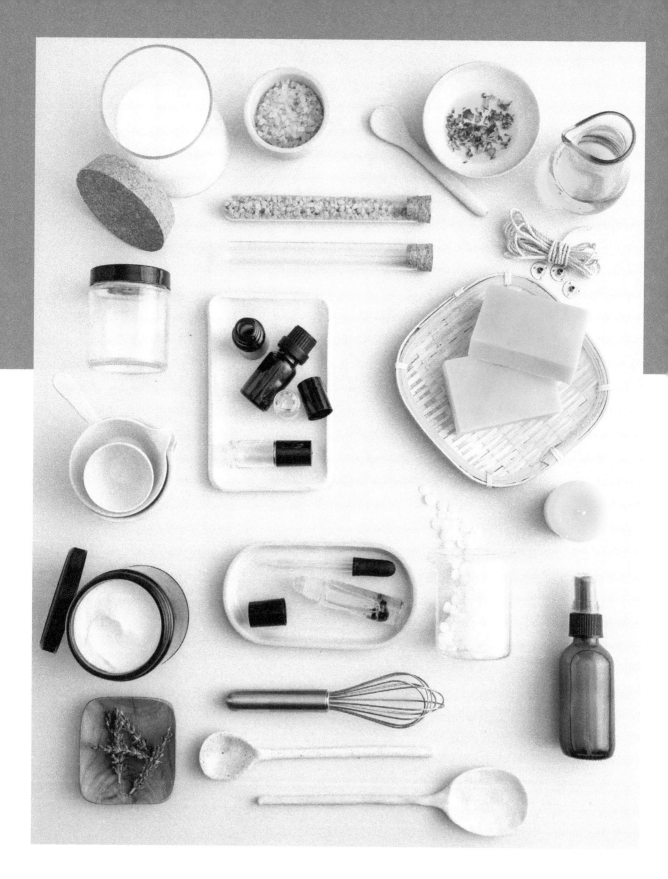

02

Your Aromatherapy Tool Kit

A lot of information on aromatherapy and essential oils exists out there—and it can quickly become overwhelming. But do not worry! In this chapter, I am going to show you that you do not have to be a chemist or spend a ton of money to get started using essential oils for self-care. I will tell you exactly what you will need to get started, what to look for when buying essential oils, and how to practice aromatherapy safely and mindfully.

SHOPPING FOR ESSENTIAL OILS

When it comes to products that your body is getting up close and personal with, quality is key. Not all essential oils are created equally, and there are some important factors to keep in mind when shopping for essential oils. Let's take a look.

What to Look For

While it is easy to find high-quality essential oils online and in stores, it is also important to know how to look for them—especially when there's a lot of confusing (and sometimes misleading) information out there. Here are some things to keep in mind.

MARKETING CLAIMS

You'll see a lot of claims being thrown around by different companies. Here's how to tell which ones you can trust:

PURITY: The label should tell you whether the oil is pure or diluted with a carrier oil. If the essential oil is not labeled, beware: It could be cut with cheaper chemicals, diluted with a carrier oil, or contain a different plant species altogether.

AROMATHERAPY GRADE OR THERAPEUTIC GRADE: Essential oils are not regulated by the US Food and Drug Administration (FDA). No official grading system or oversight process exists for the production of essential oils; instead, the manufacturing companies set their own standards for quality, so these claims do not carry too much weight—they are usually created by marketing teams.

CERTIFIED: There is also no official certification process for essential oils. Manufacturing companies may have internal certification processes, but these have no bearing on the comparable quality of essential oils produced by other companies. Again, do not put too much faith here.

READING THE LABEL

Avoid purchasing oils from companies that do not properly label their essential oils. A quality essential oil label should list the following:

- Common name of the plant from which the oil was extracted (like "rose")
- Scientific name of the plant (genus and species, usually located beneath the common name or in the ingredients list and written in Latin, like "*Rosa damascena*")
- Purity ("100 percent pure" should be listed if it is a single-source oil)
- Ingredients (only a single essential oil or a blend of essential oils should be listed)
- Directions for use and safety information

One note about **PLANT NAMES:** Occasionally, more than one version of a scientific or common name is used to designate a single plant species or subspecies used to create essential oils. Companies may combine several subspecies to create a single essential oil, as all of these plants have similar healing properties and nearly identical fragrances; for example, one reputable brand of frankincense lists three different subspecies of *Boswellia*.

Plant names also sometimes change over time as botanists reclassify plants. This book lists the most accurate scientific names at the time of printing, but if you find that a scientific name does not always exactly match what is on a product label, that does not necessarily mean you should avoid it. Do, however, pay reasonable attention to labeling and descriptions and try to buy only high-quality products from reputable manufacturers to reduce the risk of purchasing adulterated or even fake essential oils.

In addition to reading the label, you should "read" the bottle itself. Essential oils are corrosive to most types of plastic and are susceptible to oxygen, sunlight, and heat. It is best to avoid essential oils packaged in clear glass and plastic containers, even if those containers are dark-colored. And the highest-quality essential oils with the longest shelf life will come packaged in amber or blue glass bottles.

Popular Essential Oil Brands

These are some of the most popular essential oil brands out there. I recommend using this list as a starting point for your shopping research!

Aura Cacia
PROS: Wide selection of single and blended essential oils.
Affordable.
CONS: Fewer options than some other brands.

doTERRA
PROS: Extensive catalogue of single and blended essential oils.
Interactive customer service experience.
Wholesale pricing available with membership.
CONS: More expensive than other companies.

Eden Botanicals
PROS: Extensive catalogue of single and blended essential oils.
Robust returns program.
Low-cost samples are available.
Several size options are available.
CONS: More expensive than other companies.

Mountain Rose Herbs
PROS: Wide selection of ethically-sourced, organic essential oils.
Company has a good selection of bottles, tools, and ingredients.
CONS: No blends available.
More expensive than other companies.

NOW Foods Essential Oils

PROS: Good selection of the most popular essential oils.
Relatively low prices.

CONS: Fewer options than some other brands.

Plant Guru

PROS: Extensive selection of single and blended essential oils.
Several value packs and starter kits.
Lower prices than many other companies.
A wide selection of bottles, tools, and ingredients.

CONS: Only available online.

Plant Therapy

PROS: Good selection of organic essential oils.
Kid-safe organic essential oils.

CONS: More expensive than other companies.
Safety information isn't as detailed.

Rocky Mountain Oils

PROS: Extensive catalogue of single and blended essential oils.
Robust customer satisfaction policy.

CONS: More expensive than other companies.

Starwest Botanicals

PROS: Good selection of single and blended essential oils.
Competitively priced.
A good selection of bottles, tools, and ingredients.

CONS: Most products are only available online.

Young Living

PROS: Extensive catalogue of single and blended essential oils.
Interactive customer service experience.

CONS: Among the more expensive brands.

Ethical Sourcing

As essential oils grow in popularity, plants are being harvested on a larger scale, often at the cost of wild plant populations. Essential oils that are produced from plants grown organically are more expensive, but they promote sustainable practices and also tend to be more potent. Buying organic also ensures that the powerful plant extracts you are inhaling or applying topically do not contain harmful, synthetic pesticides.

I also recommend researching where the essential oil originates. Some companies harvest and sell essential oils of plants that are endangered, so knowing more information about where and how the plant grew will help you make more informed decisions and ensure that we will all be able to benefit from these amazing plants for years to come. Be an informed consumer and do not hesitate to reach out to companies to ask about their policies. Companies that invest in sustainable harvest practices tend to be the most transparent and eager to share that information with their customers.

Affordability

Essential oils can get quite pricey. This is particularly true if you focus on quality rather than affordability. For example, organic essential oils typically come at higher prices than their conventional counterparts. It is a good idea to shop around and research prices for the essential oils you are considering. This gives you a feel for the average cost of a certain quantity of the oil in question, and it helps you weed out potential imposters. Be very suspicious of essential oils that are priced far below market average since it is likely that they are either not pure or of low quality.

When you compare prices, make sure that you are comparing similarly sized bottles and that you are looking at the same plant species. For example, several different types of eucalyptus exist, and of these, *Eucalyptus globulus* is the most common as well as the least expensive species. Oils made from *Eucalyptus radiata* and *Eucalyptus citriodora* (or more accurately, *Corymbia citriodora*—lemon eucalyptus) are usually a touch pricier.

Sourcing and production methods are other factors to consider, and these can impact price as well. Again, using eucalyptus as an example, much of the world's *Eucalyptus globulus* supply now comes from farms in India and China, where production costs are lower. Organic *Eucalyptus globulus* essential oil from Australian farms typically costs more.

If you would like to try an expensive essential oil such as rose, jasmine, or neroli, but the cost is prohibitive, many of the top manufacturers offer prediluted oils, which put these incredible scents within easier reach and allows you to apply these essential oils straight out of the bottle. In this case, it is okay that the essential oil is not 100 percent pure because a quality carrier oil has been used.

Building Your Essential Collection

It's a good idea to start small in every aspect of life. Starting small while building your essential oil collection will allow you to get to know each oil and how it affects you first before you begin to blend it with others. You might find that you "click" with certain oils better than others. When you consider which oils to buy first, think about which issues you would like to address and then move forward from there. Review the healing properties on pages 66–73 to get an idea of what each essential oil helps with. Then consider things like affordability, versatility, and shelf life (some essential oils have a shorter life than others, and it is best to use your essential oils while they are fresh).

TOOLS AND EQUIPMENT

If you are new to aromatherapy and want to get started right away, all you really need are two things: essential oils and carrier oils, which you will learn about next. But once you are ready to start making the remedies in part 2, you will need some extra equipment to make that happen. You will be happy to know that you probably have most of this equipment in your kitchen already—metal or glass mixing bowls, measuring spoons, and measuring cups. You may want to invest in some separate tools just for aromatherapy at a later time, but for now, you can let your existing kitchen items pull double duty.

Carrier Oils

Carrier oils are used to dilute essential oils. This prevents them from irritating your skin. There are many different types available; here are a few of the most popular:

AVOCADO OIL: You can make your massage oils rich by adding a little nutrient-laden avocado oil. This oil is very heavy and absorbs slowly; it typically has a strong fragrance, which you may or may not like.

JOJOBA OIL: This oil is more expensive than many other carrier oils, but because of its long shelf life and excellent absorption, it is an aromatherapy favorite. If you suffer from acne or have very oily skin, you might consider replacing other carrier oils with this one—or blend it with your regular carrier oil for a lighter feel. The amount of each oil to use depends on your personal preference.

LIQUID COCONUT OIL: Unlike virgin coconut oil, liquid coconut oil (also known as fractionated coconut oil) has no odor and remains in a liquid state. It penetrates very quickly and leaves just a trace of oil behind on the skin.

ROSE HIP OIL: This is another expensive carrier oil, but it is one that is well worth adding to your medicine cabinet. It is rich in vitamins A, C, and E and makes a fantastic addition to skincare products. A little goes a long way; you can blend it with other carrier oils and still reap its benefits. The amount of each oil to use depends on your personal preference.

SWEET ALMOND OIL: Sourced from almond kernels, this oil offers a very light, nutty fragrance. It absorbs quickly and leaves just a trace of oil behind on the skin.

Tools for Blending and Storing

Because most types of plastic degrade after long-term contact with essential oils, you will want to use metal or glass tools and containers with few exceptions. Certain bottles, lip balm tubes, and jars that are sold by essential oil companies specifically for storing oils long-term are okay to use.

DARK-COLORED GLASS BOTTLES. You will always need empty glass bottles when mixing and storing undiluted essential oil blends. You can purchase special dark-colored essential oil bottles online. (To reuse a bottle and remove any oily residue, fill it with Epsom salts and then rinse it out with plain water—no soap is necessary, since the salts should dissolve the residue; another option is vodka.)

FUNNELS. Mini funnels made specifically to fit essential oil bottles and larger funnels that fit quart jars help minimize spills when you transfer finished products into storage containers.

GLASS, METAL, OR CERAMIC MIXING BOWLS. It is best to have a variety of sizes of mixing bowls for holding ingredients and blending remedies.

MEASURING CUPS AND SPOONS. Glass or metal measuring cups and spoons are necessary for preparing many of the remedies in part 2. A single liquid measuring cup marked in ounce and cup increments can perform many functions.

PIPETTES. Perfect for pulling essential oils from larger wholesale-size bottles, pipettes help you measure drops precisely. Plastic pipettes should be discarded after a single use to avoid cross-contamination.

TAPE OR LABELS. You will want to carefully mark all of your aromatherapy products with permanent marker. Printed labels are nice to have, especially if you enjoy treating others to homemade aromatherapy blends.

TWEEZERS. These are essential for handling the cotton wicks inside aromatherapy inhalers.

STORAGE BAG OR BOX. A bag or box specifically designed to store essential oils offers the ideal solution for protecting them from heat and light.

WHISKS AND METAL SPOONS. These are great for blending remedies, but avoid using ones made from wood because it absorbs oil and wastes your products.

Tools for Applying

While you can simply sniff your blend or single essential oil right out of the bottle, some items make aromatherapy self-care a little easier:

DIFFUSERS. By releasing essential oils into the air, diffusers can influence your entire environment more easily than any other aromatherapy tool. There are so many types of diffusers to choose from these days, but I prefer ultrasonic ones, which use ultrasonic vibrations to transform essential oils into a mist and disperse it into the air. Look for one with timed on/off settings to make overexposure unlikely. Be sure to clean your diffuser according to its instructions; a quick wipe with a paper towel between uses can prevent oils—especially citrus ones—from causing any erosion of surfaces.

Another option is a reed diffuser, which uses wooden sticks or reeds to absorb essential oils, pulling the scent from the bottle and allowing it to evaporate in the air. This is a great method that does not require electricity or battery power.

INHALERS. Aromatherapy inhalers, which you sniff from, are really useful when you are on the go. They are inexpensive and do not take up much space so you can carry them in your bag or even your pocket. These can be purchased in bulk and many are reusable.

JEWELRY. If you wear jewelry, you may enjoy adding an aromatherapy pendant or bracelet to your collection. These typically include a porous stone that absorbs the essential oil. Combined with the heat of your skin, this creates a diffuser-like effect. Be sure to do a sensitivity test before using an essential oil for this purpose (see page 32).

ROLLER BOTTLES. Glass roller bottles make topical application a breeze. These containers are wonderful for taking a variety of blends on the go.

SPRAY TOPS. Some of the self-care remedies in part 2 call for spray tops for your essential oil bottles, which make it easy to spray the blend onto your sheets, in the air, or on an area of your body.

Tools and Ingredients for Personal Care

If you want to make your own personal-care products, you will need additional tools and ingredients. Many of these ingredients can be purchased at the supermarket whereas others can be found online or at health food stores. This is not an exhaustive list, but it will help you stock up so you are ready to make a variety of the remedies in part 2.

ESSENTIAL TOOLS

DOUBLE BOILER. This is an excellent tool for melting waxes and butters to create your own skin creams.

GLASS JARS. These are great for storing your balms, creams, and scrubs. Mason jars are inexpensive, come in a variety of sizes, and work great. Make sure to store your jars in a cool, dark place for the best shelf life.

LIP BALM FILLING TRAY. If you want to make lots of lip balm and store it in handy tubes, you will love how a filling tray makes the process quick, simple, and relatively mess-free.

MIXER. A handheld or stand mixer is good for whipping up rich body creams and blending big batches of a product.

SPECIALTY CONTAINERS. Items such as tins, lip balm tubes, and cosmetics jars give your products a beautiful, finished look. (There is no need to worry about metal or other container interactions with these, as the essential oils are so diluted at this point that it does not matter so much.)

HELPFUL INGREDIENTS

BAKING SODA. Some body-care remedies and household cleaners call for this basic ingredient. Buy a big box and get ready to have fun with it.

BEESWAX. Beeswax stiffens balms beautifully while sealing in moisture. You can use a vegan alternative if you prefer—candelilla wax, carnauba wax, and organic soy wax are suitable stand-ins.

BUTTERS. Shea and cocoa butters are essential for making thick, rich body butters that offer great hydration. Each has a distinct texture and odor, so try them out to find what you like best.

EPSOM SALTS. Many remedies call for a soothing aromatherapy bath. Epsom salts help absorb oils, making them the perfect medium for getting essential oils into your bath without worrying about skin irritation or leaving an oily ring behind.

UNSCENTED BODYWASH, SHAMPOO, CONDITIONER, AND LOTION. While you can create your own basic, unscented body-care products, for simplicity, this book makes extensive use of unscented bases. These are least expensive when purchased online in bulk.

VIRGIN COCONUT OIL. Often a substitute for shortening in your kitchen, this is fantastic for oil pulling (if you do not know what that is, see page 175). It is also used in other dental health remedies and makes its way into a variety of balms and moisturizers.

WITCH HAZEL. This herbal tonic lets you make lovely skin toners, refreshing body sprays, and other products. It is inexpensive and very easy to find at drugstores and most supermarkets. Look for the alcohol-free variety, which will not worsen dry skin.

Skincare as Self-Care?

Taking care of yourself goes way deeper than your facial mask, but that does not mean there is not a place for skincare in self-care. In fact, Jennifer Wolkin, a psychologist at the Joan H. Tisch Center for Women's Health at NYU Langone Medical Center, commented on skincare rituals as a "way to create a sense of control," thereby "decreasing negative thoughts or reducing uncertainty to create an illusion of control." So, your skincare ritual can actually be helping with your anxiety, too. By using essential oils, you are using ingredients that help both your skin and mind feel clear.

Whether you treat skincare more like a pampering session or an essential part of your daily well-being, I think we can all agree that taking time to focus on something that makes you feel good is always a bonus. Here is a relaxing skincare ritual that uses a jade roller, a paint roller-like tool for your face. Jade rollers have been around since 17th-century China, but they've recently come back into popularity, and for good reason—they feel luxurious without costing a fortune. The perfect tool for maximum relaxation!

1. Put your jade roller in the freezer for about 10 to 15 minutes before using.
2. While the jade roller is cooling, wash your face and then apply some diluted frankincense essential oil or Nourishing Rose Antiaging Serum (see page 154).

3. Get your jade roller and, starting in the center of your face, apply gentle pressure outward and upward across your face.
4. Keep rolling outward and downward on your neck, which will stimulate your lymphatic system.

The coolness of the stone will help with puffiness, the gentle rolling will help the serum penetrate further, and you will feel super relaxed!

STORAGE

Essential oils have antibacterial and antifungal properties that prevent mold or mildew growth, but they do have a shelf life that is decreased by exposure to oxygen, light, and heat. When essential oils are subjected to any of these three things over time, their chemistry changes and they are considered oxidized or "expired." Proper storage and handling are key to protecting your essential oils and maximizing their shelf life; they can last from two to five years, depending on the oil.

To avoid oxidation, always make sure that the lids on your essential oil bottles are sealed properly when not in use. Do not store essential oils in bottles with dropper caps because these caps do not fully seal, and the essential oil will eventually erode the rubber top.

Also, keep your essential oils away from light, especially sunlight. They should be stored in dark amber or blue glass bottles to protect them from UV rays. The bottles themselves should also be stored away from light in a cabinet or a lidded box. Besides darkness, keep them cool, too. I store my own essential oils in a cabinet, but they also can be stored in the refrigerator.

You can keep your essential oils in the freezer, but it does not extend their shelf life over storing them in a refrigerator. If you do freeze them, make sure your oils return to room temperature before you use them. Some oils might even crystallize when frozen. You can usually determine the shelf life of your blend by using the expiration date of the carrier oil. If your blend is also using non-oil ingredients like sugar, aloe vera, or beeswax, go by the expiration date of those ingredients.

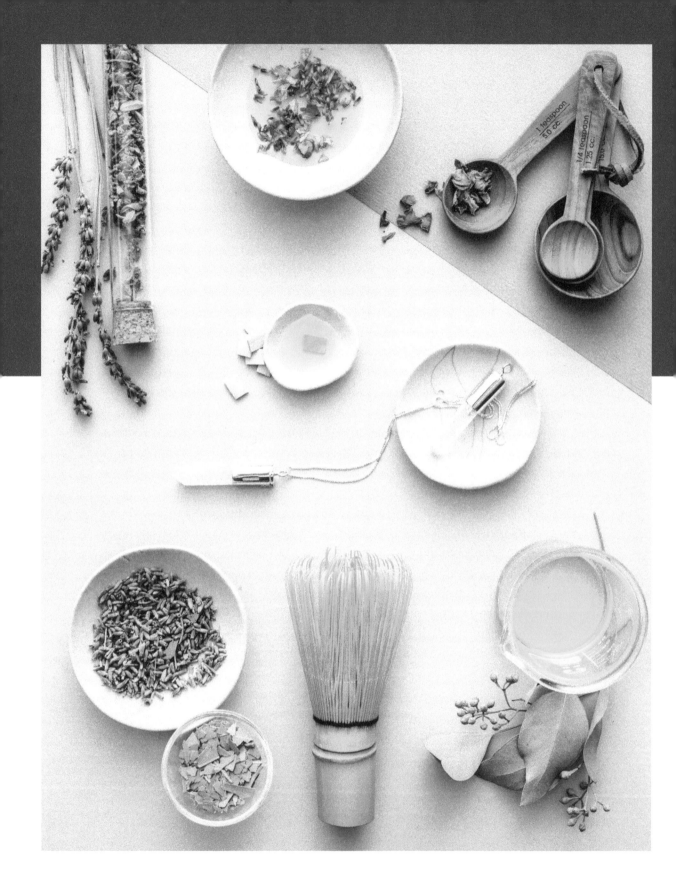

03

Using Essential Oils

There are so many wonderful ways to put your essential oils to work in your life. This chapter guides you through all of these options, including different methods of application, when to use single oils and when to use blends, and even how to start creating your own blends. You will also learn how to do all of this safely, so that you can reap the rewards of your efforts without any worry!

SAFETY AND BEST PRACTICES

Many people assume that because essential oils are natural, they cannot be harmful. As you learned from the earlier discussion on natural medicines, just because something is natural does not mean it is harmless. Essential oils are highly concentrated extracts from some of the most potent plants on the planet, and if used incorrectly, they can absolutely have negative effects. Fortunately, essential oil safety is not complicated, so by taking just a few simple precautions, you can enjoy their many benefits without concern.

Before you make a final decision about which essential oils to try first, double-check the safety information to ensure that the oils you are considering are safe for you to use. More than a few come with warnings about interactions with pharmaceuticals and most are not recommended for women who are pregnant or nursing.

Dilution

It takes an enormous amount of plant material to make just a drop of essential oil—for example, it takes about 60 roses to make a single drop of pure rose essential oil! Every drop of essential oil contains the concentrated chemical components from all the plants that went into it. These extracts do not dissolve in water and should not be used directly on the skin. This is why it is so important to dilute essential oils with a carrier oil before applying them. You can find more in-depth information about dilution later in this chapter.

Sensitivity Test

First of all, if you are allergic to certain plants or plant families, avoid all of the essential oils that come from those plants. But even if you are not allergic, some oils can cause skin reactions, especially when used "neat" (undiluted). It is always smart to conduct a patch test before trying a new essential oil. To do this, moisten a cotton ball with 3 or 4 drops of a carrier oil, add 1 drop of the essential oil to the cotton ball, and dab the cotton ball on the inner fold of your elbow. Discard the cotton ball and cover the spot with a bandage and check for irritation 24 hours later. If you notice irritation, avoid the essential oil topically; inhaling the oil should still be okay.

Practicing Mindfulness with Essential Oils

"Mindfulness" is a trendy term in the wellness world these days, and although it might sound like something that can be done only in a super-Zen setting, practicing mindfulness is all about paying attention and being in the moment—wherever you are.

Practicing mindfulness with essential oils means paying attention to how you are feeling physically, mentally, and emotionally so that you can come up with an aromatherapy self-care game plan. It is also about noticing how a particular scent or remedy changes how you feel.

Being mindful with essential oils also includes respecting the plants that provide these oils and not using them unnecessarily or in excess. As with most things, start slowly with small amounts. More does not mean better, and in fact, overdoing it can have harmful effects. Be sure to dilute essential oils whenever possible and use them with intention. Remember, you can always add additional drops of oil to your blends, but you cannot remove them. It is not just safer and more cost-effective for you—it is also better for our planet!

Always be on the lookout for other adverse reactions to oils. The most common one is skin sensitivity, but if you experience headaches or nausea after using a specific oil, it may be best to avoid that oil in the future.

Internal Ingestion

Never internally ingest essential oils without professional guidance. Ingesting multiple drops of an essential oil can eventually damage the liver, kidneys, stomach, and intestines, even if an essential oil sales representative tells you that it is safe. There is a place for ingestion in aromatherapy, but only under the supervision of a professionally certified aromatherapist and a medical practitioner. None of the remedies in this book are for internal ingestion.

Photosensitization

Some essential oils cause photosensitization, meaning that they can increase your risk of sunburn. Citrus oils are the most common essential oils that cause this because they contain compounds called furanocoumarins that increase UV sensitivity. Other oils can also contain furanocoumarins or other compounds that have the same effect, so always be sure to check the label of an oil to see if it causes photosensitivity. If you topically use an essential oil with a photosensitization warning, avoid sun exposure and tanning beds for 6 to 24 hours after application, depending on the individual essential oil and the warning that accompanies it. Here are some common citrus oils to know about:

CITRUS ESSENTIAL OILS KNOWN TO BE PHOTOTOXIC: bergamot, grapefruit, lemon (cold-pressed), lime (cold-pressed), bitter orange (cold-pressed), mandarin leaf, and clementine

NONPHOTOTOXIC CITRUS ESSENTIAL OILS: bergamot (if it is furocoumarin-free or FCF, also known as bergapten-free), lemon (steam-distilled), lemon leaf (note that this is different from lemon-peel essential oil, which is simply called "lemon"), lime (steam-distilled), mandarin, sweet orange, orange leaf, and tangelo

Pregnancy

When used properly, many essential oils are safe to use while you are pregnant, and they can help expectant mothers with difficult symptoms. If you are pregnant or breastfeeding, always discuss the use of essential oils with your health-care provider. Aromatherapists agree that most essential oils should be avoided during the first trimester of pregnancy, but it is generally safe to use them sparingly through the rest of a pregnancy with these guidelines in mind:

ALWAYS DILUTE ESSENTIAL OILS WITH A CARRIER OIL BEFORE USE. If you are pregnant, you should not exceed a 1 percent dilution or 9 drops of essential oil per ounce of carrier oil. This dilution can vary depending on the specific essential oil, so be sure to check the maximum recommended dilution for each oil to avoid irritation.

LIMIT DIFFUSION. Pregnant women are more susceptible to essential oil overexposure, and prolonged diffuser use can result in headaches, nausea, and dizziness. Therefore, the diffuser should run for only 10 to 15 minutes at a time.

MINIMIZE DAILY USE AS MUCH AS POSSIBLE. During pregnancy, it is best to use essential oils only when you need them for symptom relief.

Other Populations

Keep essential oils out of the reach of children and pets. Children under age 12, elderly people, and those with compromised immune systems are often highly sensitive to essential oils. Be cautious about overexposure and use extra care by doing a sensitivity test of the essential oils in a remedy before using it.

HOW TO APPLY

As you have learned, you can apply essential oils either topically or by inhaling them. This sounds simple enough, but there are actually tons of ways to go about both methods. I will cover all the options so that you can pick and choose what works best for you.

Inhalation

Inhaling essential oils is the fastest method of getting essential oils into the bloodstream, as they travel into your brain, lungs, and circulatory system. Here are some of the most commonly used inhalation applications:

DIFFUSERS. Diffusing essential oils is passive inhalation and can provide overall benefit by reducing stress, uplifting mood, and assisting in a restful night's sleep. Because essential oils are powerful and work quickly, diffusing for short times is preferred over diffusing for hours. Keep in mind that everyone in the vicinity of the diffuser will be inhaling the essential oil along with you, so be sure that others are okay with this before you use one.

HUMIDIFIER. If you have a cold-mist humidifier, it should be able to safely handle essential oils. Check with your humidifier's manufacturer to make sure that the oils will not damage the machine.

INHALERS. Aromatherapy inhalers are available in plastic or a combination of glass and metal, and they have many benefits over a diffuser. While a diffuser exposes everyone in the immediate area to the aroma, an aromatherapy inhaler is user-specific—that is, it is just for you. Inhalers are discreet and portable (plastic ones look a lot like a tube of lip balm), so you can take them with you wherever you go. For example, if you get overwhelmed in public spaces, you can grab your inhaler and sniff your way to calm. Aromatherapy jewelry works in much the same way and is a fun, fashionable option.

SHOWER STEAMER. All it takes is a couple of drops of essential oil on a washcloth or a shower steamer (similar to bath bombs) to enjoy a relaxing "getaway." Steam is especially helpful for respiratory issues.

SPRAY FOR BODY AND ROOM. Sprays can effectively disperse essential oils on your body, clothing, bed linens, or furniture and can provide an alternative to dangerous and sometimes toxic synthetic room fragrances.

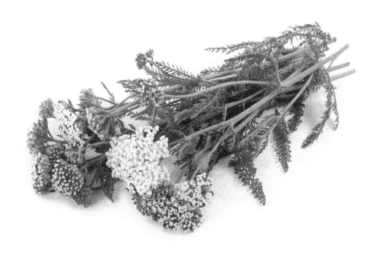

Using Acupressure with Essential Oils

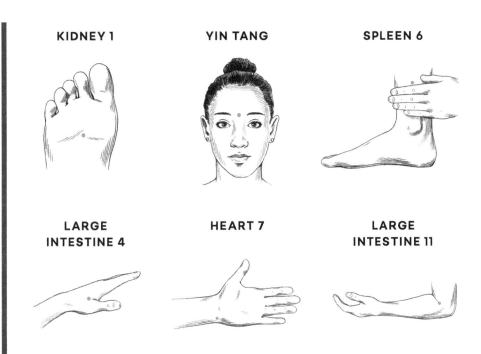

KIDNEY 1

YIN TANG

SPLEEN 6

LARGE INTESTINE 4

HEART 7

LARGE INTESTINE 11

As an acupuncturist, I often recommend that my patients apply essential oils to acupressure points at home. If you need some quick grounding, rub a few drops of diluted lavender oil onto Kidney 1 and Heart 7. If you're feeling anxious, use a drop of diluted frankincense oil on Yin Tang. For headaches, try diluted peppermint oil on Large Intestine 4. For allergies or fevers, a few drops of diluted peppermint oil on Large Intestine 11 (located at the outside of the elbow crease) works wonders. For menstrual cramps, try a few drops of diluted clary sage oil on Spleen 6 (located four finger widths above the ankle bone).

Topical

For topical applications, essential oils are diluted with a carrier oil and then applied directly to the skin. This type of application is the slowest method of getting essential oils into the bloodstream. Applying diluted essential oil this way has many wellness benefits, but it is most beneficial when you are treating the skin itself. These are some of the most commonly used methods of topical applications:

BATHS. Aromatic baths are used for everything from muscle pains to cold and flu symptoms. A relaxing bath with essential oils can lift a depressed mood and reduce stress.

HAIRCARE PRODUCTS. Essential oils can be used to lengthen, strengthen, and detoxify your hair and scalp. When added to shampoo, they can stop dandruff and even repel and kill head lice.

HOT AND COLD COMPRESSES. In place of a bath, hot or cold compresses can be very helpful when body temperatures spike or you need to reduce anxiety. Compresses can also be used to clean certain wounds.

LOTIONS, CREAMS, AND BODY BUTTERS. Essential oils in these products can target wrinkles, fine lines, scars, dry skin, and cellulite.

MASSAGE OILS. Probably the oldest method of topical application, an aromatherapy massage can heal tired muscles and calm anxious minds.

ROLLERBALL BOTTLES. Beyond applying a diluted oil or blend directly to your skin using your fingertips, a rollerball is the easiest method of topical application.

SALVES AND BALMS. Used to heal cuts, scrapes, and abrasions, these aromatherapy products can also help with acute issues such as muscle pain, menstrual cramps, and growing pains.

VAPOR RUBS. Certain essential oils added to a vapor rub for your chest can help alleviate coughs, congestion, and stuffy noses.

SINGLE OILS VERSUS BLENDS

When you shop for essential oils, you will notice that you can purchase single oils or blends. What is the difference? And which ones are right for you?

SINGLE OILS. A single essential oil is the extract of one plant and nothing else. Each single oil is made up of its own complex combination of natural elements that work together to provide certain benefits. As you learn about aromatherapy, it is best to focus first on single oils to get a deeper understanding of their individual properties before buying blends. All the remedies in part 2 call for single essential oils that you will combine into blends yourself.

BLENDS. Essential oil blends are a synergistic combination of two or more single essential oils for a purpose greater than and different from any one individual oil. Aromatherapists create unique blends to target specific needs. While you can purchase premixed essential oil blends (which often come with nifty names), it can be cheaper and more effective in the long run to purchase single essential oils and blend them to suit your own needs. Part 2 will get you started.

Single oils and blends are both great tools for using aromatherapy for self-care. Using single oils helps you figure out how different oils affect you—you might experience skin irritation from a particular oil when applied topically or discover that an oil is too potent for you. You may find that an essential oil intended to be calming has an energizing effect on you instead. Making your own blends allows you to start combining single oils that you like for more powerful and targeted results.

Creating Your Own Blends

In part 2, you will find 100 great blends to start using right away, but once you begin to get the hang of the process, you can create your own customized blends for your self-care needs. The first question you will want to ask is: What's the purpose? Defining your goal will help you select a method to create your blend. For instance, to make a blend to help you sleep better, you would select essential oils with calming and relaxing properties and then decide which type of application would suit you and your issue best.

How do you go about blending? Well, in general, essential oils from the same category (citrus, floral, herbal, or spice) tend to blend well with one another. You cannot go wrong with a blend of lemon and grapefruit, for example, or a combination of peppermint and rosemary. Citrus and spice essential oils tend to complement one another beautifully, as do herbs and citrus; for example, many people enjoy the classic combination of lemon and peppermint.

How many oils are too many to blend together? Well, the number depends. If your goal is to create a therapeutic blend but have a pleasant scent, three to five oils are ideal. If your main goal is therapeutic benefits, the scent might be less important, so you can safely mix more than five. (Be sure to keep notes on your blends so that you can make them again or modify them later.)

When blending, you will want to add your essential oils to one another, allow them to mingle for a time, and then add the carrier oil. Letting them "rest"—for as little as 1 hour or up to 2 or 3 days—creates synergy and gives the aroma a chance to fully develop. Keep your empty (and clean) essential oil bottles for this purpose—it is cheaper for you and better for the earth!

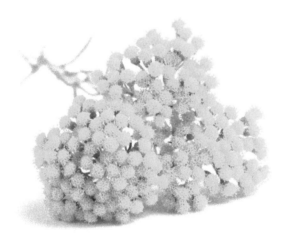

A Handy Blending Formula

Similar to a perfume, essential oil blends also have different aromatic notes. Following this formula is not always necessary, but if scent is very important to you, make sure every blend has one or more of each of these notes.

TOP NOTES: Top notes are often the first noticeable aromas in a blend but also the aromas that evaporate the quickest. These include all citrus oils, basil, eucalyptus, lavender, peppermint, and spearmint.

MIDDLE NOTES: Middle notes are sometimes referred to as the heart or the center of an aromatherapy blend. Their aromas will last a little longer than top notes on a perfume blotter or your skin. These include chamomile, cinnamon, clary sage, clove bud, fir, geranium, sweet marjoram, black pepper, rose, rosemary, tea tree, and thyme.

BASE NOTES: The base notes stick around the longest on a perfume blotter or your skin. If the oil is thick enough, it will hold on to the middle and top notes a little bit longer. These notes include cedarwood, frankincense, ginger, sandalwood, vanilla, and vetiver.

DILUTION

Regardless of how you choose to use essential oils topically, dilution is the key to safe and effective use. Never apply a "neat" or undiluted essential oil directly to the skin without using a carrier oil. By using just a single drop of any essential oil neat on the skin, you risk developing a permanent sensitization to that oil and you will miss out on its benefits in the future.

Diluting essential oils is as simple as combining them with a carrier oil. The dilution percentage depends on the type of application, the person, and their age. The basic dilution chart on page 42 is handed out in aromatherapy classes, but keep in mind that this is a general reference chart for blends. Some essential oils require more dilution than others, so when you start experimenting with essential oils on your own, be sure to research each one to see what dilution percentage is recommended to prevent potential reactions.

To research this, *Essential Oil Safety: A Guide for Health Care Professionals* by Robert Tisserand and Rodney Young is the definitive authority—nothing else even comes close. It is available both as a print book and e-book. It contains 400 highly detailed essential oil profiles (including some unusual ones) and it covers drug interactions, which is very helpful for anyone who takes pharmaceuticals.

Those who do not feel like investing in an entire book on essential oil safety might find Tisserand's downloadable dilution chart useful, but quite general. Tisserand's website does offer some specific cautions and plenty of good information geared toward better overall safety (see Resources on page 188).

Last but not least, people who want to take a deep dive into aromatherapy might consider continuing education. The National Association for Holistic Aromatherapy (NAHA) has a list of schools, and of those, quite a few offer online courses (see Resources on page 188).

DILUTION CHART

CARRIER OIL IN OUNCES	0.5%	1%	1.5%	2.5%	3%	5%	10%
½ OUNCE	1 to 2 drops	3 drops	5 drops	7 to 8 drops	9 drops	15 drops	30 drops
1 OUNCE	3 drops	6 drops	9 drops	15 drops	18 drops	30 drops	60 drops
2 OUNCES	6 drops	12 drops	24 drops	30 drops	36 drops	60 drops	120 drops

DILUTION %	USES
0.5%	Babies, frail or elderly individuals
1%	Babies, children, pregnant and nursing mothers, frail or elderly individuals
1.5%	Subtle aromatherapy, emotional and energetic work, frail or elderly individuals, face creams, lotions, exfoliants
2.5% TO 3%	Massage oils, general skincare, lotions, facial oils, body oils, body butter
5%	Treatment massages, acute treatment, wound healing, healing salves, body butter
10%	Muscular aches and pains, trauma injury, treatment massage, acute physical pain, salves and balms

SUBSTITUTION

With so many essential oils out there (some of them quite expensive), here is a popular question: When and what can I substitute? While this can sometimes be as easy as using a similarly scented oil, that might not always work for your goal. Here are three different methods you can use to choose a substitute essential oil for any remedy:

AROMATIC SUBSTITUTIONS. If scent is your goal, substitute with essential oils from the same family. Scent families include citrusy, woodsy, earthy, floral, spicy, minty, and medicinal.

THERAPEUTIC SUBSTITUTIONS. If you have therapeutic goals, substitute with essential oils with the same or similar healing properties. Spearmint is a common substitution for peppermint, for example. It is less potent but provides similar effects, such as relief from nausea and indigestion.

CHEMICAL SIMILARITIES. Chemistry is ultimately what gives an essential oil its therapeutic properties. This is a more advanced method of substitution, and if you are interested in learning more, check out the book *Essential Oil Safety: A Guide for Health Care Professionals* by Robert Tisserand and Rodney Young. As a quick example, 1,8-cineole is a healing component found in helichrysum, eucalyptus, and several other essential oils that can be used interchangeably for their analgesic, anti-inflammatory, and antibacterial properties. Even though these essential oils offer different aromas, they provide similar benefits.

If a remedy in part 2 lists an essential oil that you do not have in your aromatherapy collection, you can substitute it for any of the alternates I recommend in the next chapter. Read on!

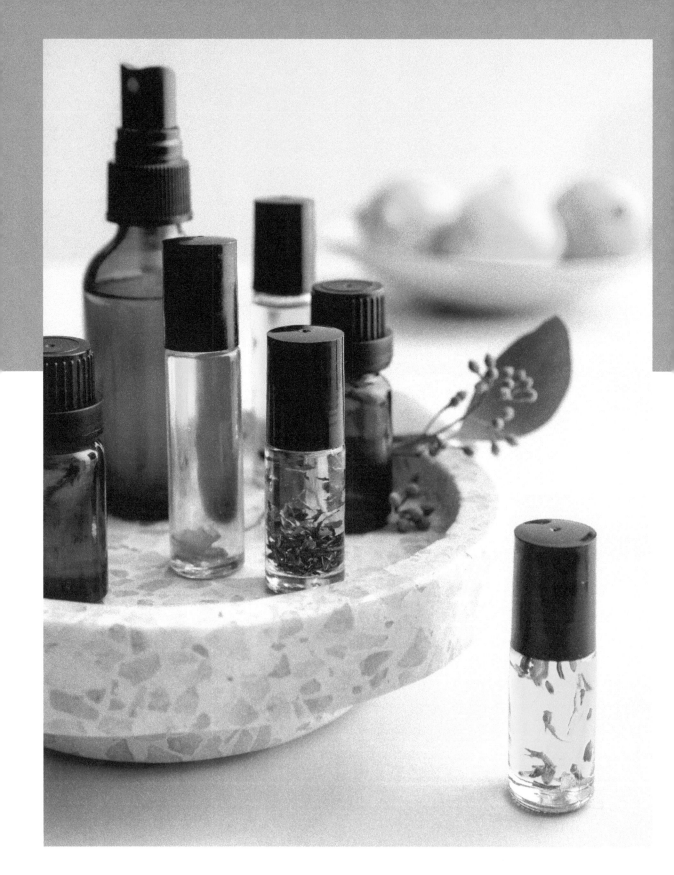

04

Go-To Essential Oils for Self-Care

Nature's abundant pharmacy offers more than 300 essential oils. If this sounds a bit overwhelming, you will be happy to know that this book focuses on just 50 of the most versatile oils. Each essential oil included here provides mental, emotional, and physical benefits. Together, this collection of essential oils makes up a full self-care package.

If you are just getting started, I recommend 10 must-haves for overall well-being. Each one of these top 10 essential oils is highly versatile, offering a lot of bang for your buck. You'll find profiles for all 10 in this chapter, followed by a chart that includes information on the remaining 40 oils used in this book. This chart is a great reference tool to use when you start building your collection!

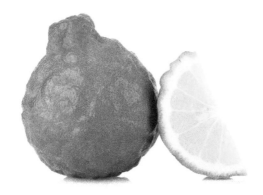

Bergamot
(Citrus bergamia)

If you have ever enjoyed the delicious aroma of a steaming cup of Earl Grey tea, then you have already been introduced to bergamot. Complex floral notes lie beneath this oil's citrusy tang; in fact, its scent reminds many people of the cheery scent of orange. Bergamot's uplifting fragrance soothes frayed nerves, eases anxiety, and lifts misery's clouds. Carefully diluted, it comforts itchy skin and helps clear up blemishes.

SAFETY PRECAUTIONS

According to *Essential Oil Safety: A Guide for Health Care Professionals* by Robert Tisserand and Rodney Young, cold-pressed bergamot essential oil is phototoxic and should be topically applied at a maximum dilution of 0.4 percent. Choosing a bergapten-free version reduces phototoxicity.

SUBSTITUTES

Lemon, mandarin, sweet orange

BLENDS WELL WITH

Lavender, patchouli, clary sage, cypress, lime, frankincense, jasmine

HEALING PROPERTIES

1. Aids in relaxation
2. Antibiotic
3. Antidepressant
4. Helps control infection
5. Helps prevent cramping and muscle spasms
6. Promotes digestion
7. Promotes healing and the formation of healthy scar tissue
8. Reduces fever
9. Relieves pain

USES

Bergamot essential oil supports energy while also easing tension. Its ability to simultaneously relax the mind and uplift the senses makes it an excellent antidote to life's stresses. Topically, bergamot can help produce even skin tone by fading dark spots and softening scars. This property, paired with its uplifting scent, makes it a nice addition to your favorite hand cream.

- Add a few drops of bergamot essential oil to your diffuser when you are feeling stressed.
- Mix 1 drop bergamot with 1 tablespoon unscented shower gel for a relaxing, uplifting aromatherapy experience in the shower.
- Try the Uplifting Diffuser Blend (see page 81) for depression.

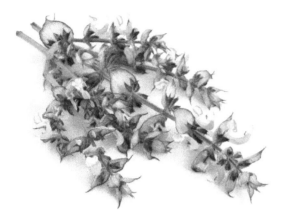

Clary sage
(Salvia sclarea)

Clary sage essential oil offers a warm, distinctly herbaceous fragrance with a slightly floral undernote and plenty of earthy richness. Soothing and grounding, this essential oil is one of the best for insomnia. Clary sage is beneficial for menstrual cramps and hot flashes, and it supports hormonal balance. Its pain-relieving properties make it useful for a variety of concerns, including sore muscles and headaches. Clary sage can help restore emotional stability in times of nervousness, anxiety, and stress.

SAFETY PRECAUTIONS

Clary sage is a strong *emmenagogue*, meaning that it can stimulate menstruation; it is not for use during pregnancy. The estrogen-like action of clary sage makes this essential oil one to use cautiously if you are at a high risk for breast cancer. Numerous sources recommend avoiding clary sage when driving due to its strong relaxation properties.

SUBSTITUTES

Lavender, Roman chamomile

BLENDS WELL WITH

Lavender, lemon, fennel, frankincense, mandarin, cedarwood, rose geranium

HEALING PROPERTIES

1. Aids in sleep and deep relaxation
2. Antibacterial
3. Antidepressant
4. Helps control infection
5. Helps prevent cramping and muscle spasms
6. Lowers blood pressure
7. Reduces gas and supports healthy digestion
8. Stimulates or promotes menstruation

USES

Clary sage essential oil encourages balance on so many levels. Intensely calming, it provides a grounding presence in diffuser blends for stress, insomnia, and tension. Applied topically in a massage oil, it offers soothing relief from a variety of physical discomforts. Feel content, relaxed, and at ease with clary sage essential oil.

- Ease anxiety and lift your spirits by diffusing clary sage.
- Use 4 drops in 1 teaspoon of carrier oil to create a soothing bath for cramps, muscle pain, PMS, or menopause symptoms.
- Try the Dreamtime Pillow Spray (see page 140).

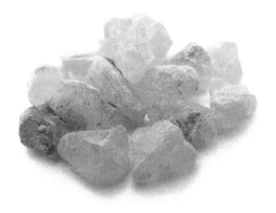

Frankincense
(Boswellia sacra)

Frankincense is well known for its ability to calm the senses and restore inner peace. It is often used to create meditative blends that play up its spicy, woody fragrance while grounding the mind and reducing mental chatter. As wonderful as its scent is, there is more to this versatile oil than just what meets the nose. It heals, rejuvenates, and balances even the most troubled skin, making it a great addition to lotions, cleansers, and other topical applications.

SAFETY PRECAUTIONS

Frankincense is generally regarded as safe.

SUBSTITUTES

Myrrh, sandalwood

BLENDS WELL WITH

Myrrh, lavender, geranium, Roman chamomile, vetiver, ylang-ylang

HEALING PROPERTIES

1. Aids in sleep and deep relaxation
2. Astringent
3. Energizing and strengthening
4. Helps control infection
5. Promotes healing and the formation of healthy scar tissue
6. Promotes urination
7. Reduces gas
8. Stimulates or promotes menstruation
9. Supports healthy digestion
10. Thins mucus

USES

Frankincense is often referred to as the king of oils and for good reason. At the top of the list of its benefits is its ability to calm the mind, ease anxiety, and create a sense of inner stillness. Frankincense gently eases congestion and opens up the respiratory system. It soothes inflamed skin and helps heal minor wounds, and in some cases, it can even reduce the appearance of scars. For mind, body, and spirit, frankincense is a definite must-have.

- Add a few drops to your diffuser to soothe cold symptoms.
- Rejuvenate facial skin with a 1:1 combination of frankincense and your favorite carrier oil. Apply a few drops once or twice daily.
- Try the Inspire Inner Vision Diffuser Blend (see page 122) for boosting creativity.

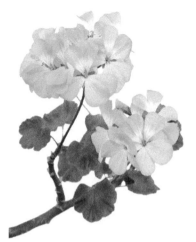

Geranium
(Pelargonium graveolens)

With its fresh, green aroma, geranium offers a touch of floral sweetness and the barest hints of apple and mint. Cheerful and uplifting, it eases negativity and quickly banishes the blues while imparting a sense of good-natured balance. Topically, it is among the best for soothing compromised skin.

SAFETY PRECAUTIONS

Not recommended for use during pregnancy or while breastfeeding.

SUBSTITUTES

Rose geranium

BLENDS WELL WITH

Orange, lemon, rose, Roman chamomile, patchouli, basil, bergamot

HEALING PROPERTIES

1. Antidepressant
2. Astringent
3. Encourages wound healing
4. Energizing and strengthening
5. Helps control infection
6. Helps slow or stop minor bleeding
7. Promotes healing and the formation of healthy scar tissue
8. Promotes urination
9. Relieves pain
10. Stimulates cellular growth or regeneration

USES

Ancient Egyptians used geranium to promote smooth, radiant skin and you can do the same. A great remedy for oily skin, geranium is also excellent for soothing itchy conditions like eczema. Its antibacterial and antifungal properties make it a useful addition to acne remedies, and its ability to ease inflammation makes it helpful in massage oils for cramps, aches, and pains. While enjoying geranium's many external applications, you might also notice that it brings a sense of refreshed, balanced calm to your mind.

- Feeling overwhelmed? Add geranium essential oil to your diffuser to alleviate stress, tension, anxiety, or anger.
- Add 1 drop to your morning moisturizer to smooth, heal, and balance facial skin.
- Make a delightful body spray with 12 drops geranium essential oil mixed into ⅓ cup water and 1 tablespoon witch hazel. This simple remedy doubles as a natural insect repellent.
- Try the Soothing PMS Massage Oil (see page 176) to restore balance during your monthly cycle.

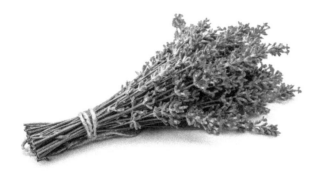

Lavender
(Lavandula angustifolia)

Lavender's peaceful, enticing aroma balances floral and herbal notes like nothing else. Renowned for its ability to promote tranquil sleep while alleviating stress and anxiety, lavender can help ease emotional trauma and tension, too. This essential oil is a must for skin irritation, and its ability to soothe headaches, sore muscles, and deeper joint pain makes it a favorite for much more than simply creating a calm environment.

SAFETY PRECAUTIONS

Lavender essential oil is generally considered safe.

SUBSTITUTES

Spike lavender, lavandin

BLENDS WELL WITH

Lemon, eucalyptus, rosemary, sage, thyme, peppermint

HEALING PROPERTIES

1. Aids in sleep and deep relaxation
2. Anti-inflammatory
3. Antibacterial
4. Antidepressant
5. Fights viral infections
6. Helps prevent cramping and muscle spasms
7. Lowers blood pressure
8. Promotes healing and the formation of healthy scar tissue
9. Reduces gas
10. Relieves pain

USES

Lavender essential oil helps restore calm in almost any situation involving tension, nervousness, panic, or anxiety. It can help you push your reset button by promoting restful sleep, and when you are headachy or feeling sore, its pain-relieving effect brings relief, particularly when paired with a soothing massage. Skin problems are no match for lavender: Try it for acne, minor wounds and burns, sunburn, and insect bites. For congestion, simply inhale and enjoy clearer breathing.

- Diffuse lavender in your home to promote a sense of calm while freshening air naturally.
- Support overall well-being by adding 4 or 5 drops lavender essential oil and 1 teaspoon carrier oil to a warm bath.
- Soothe sore muscles by blending 4 drops lavender essential oil with 1 tablespoon of your favorite carrier oil for a relaxing massage.
- Try Soothing After-Sun Balm (see page 180) to help heal the effects of overexposure to UV rays.

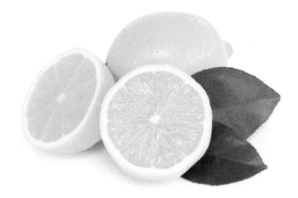

Lemon
(Citrus limon)

Crisp and refreshing, the scent of lemon essential oil is unmistakable. This fragrance soothes, uplifts, and nurtures, particularly in times of emotional upset. When you are feeling good, you will find that the invigorating scent of lemon enhances and intensifies positive emotions. This oil is an excellent one to diffuse anytime you need a physical or mental energy boost.

SAFETY PRECAUTIONS

According to *Essential Oil Safety: A Guide for Health Care Professionals* by Robert Tisserand and Rodney Young, cold-pressed lemon essential oil is phototoxic whereas steam-distilled lemon oil is not. If you choose cold-pressed lemon essential oil, the maximum dilution rate for topical application is 2 percent (see page 42).

SUBSTITUTES

Mandarin, lime, grapefruit

BLENDS WELL WITH

Clove, grapefruit, mandarin, orange, cinnamon, rosemary, thyme

HEALING PROPERTIES

1. Antibacterial
2. Boosts immunity
3. Energizes and strengthens
4. Helps control infection
5. Increases circulation
6. Induces sweat
7. Lowers blood pressure
8. Promotes urination
9. Reduces fever
10. Reduces gas

USES

Since lemon essential oil can increase the risk of sunburn, it is enjoyed in aromatic applications more frequently than in topical ones, where it quickly alleviates cold and flu symptoms such as cough and congestion while simultaneously lifting your spirits. Used well-diluted and sparingly, it can help with acne, sore muscles, and skin irritation. In addition to brightening your mood, adding lemon essential oil to shampoo and conditioner can help balance oily hair.

- Feeling irritated or just plain exhausted? Try adding lemon to your diffuser for a quick pick-me-up.
- Add 3 drops lemon essential oil to 1 ounce unscented body cream for an energizing all-over moisture treatment. Avoid sun exposure with this remedy.
- Try the Enthusiasm Diffuser Blend (see page 123) next time you need an energy boost.

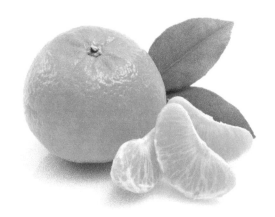

Mandarin
(Citrus × aurantium)

Irresistibly sweet and incredibly refreshing, mandarin essential oil can help you banish the blues and beat stress. Milder than other citrus essential oils, mandarin is a wonderful choice for uplifting body lotions that leave you feeling refreshed and motivated. When it is time to unwind, mandarin's lively, nurturing presence encourages you to mentally relax without promoting drowsiness.

SAFETY PRECAUTIONS

According to *Essential Oil Safety: A Guide for Health Care Professionals* by Robert Tisserand and Rodney Young, mandarin is not phototoxic but it can cause skin irritation if it becomes oxidized due to overexposure to heat and light or if moisture enters the bottle. Store it carefully and use it while fresh to prevent sensitization.

SUBSTITUTES

Lemon, lime, sweet orange

BLENDS WELL WITH

Basil, spearmint, orange, grapefruit, clove, frankincense, helichrysum

HEALING PROPERTIES

1. Aids digestion and alleviates digestive discomfort
2. Detoxifying and purifying
3. Helps control infection
4. Helps prevent cramping and muscle spasms
5. Increases circulation
6. Promotes healing and the formation of healthy scar tissue
7. Promotes the release of bile
8. Promotes urination
9. Relaxing
10. Supports healthy digestion

USES

Mandarin essential oil supports a calm, happy environment, easing nervous tension and relieving stress. Its diuretic properties make it a good remedy for bloating and water retention. If you are suffering from a digestive imbalance such as gas, constipation, or diarrhea, a gentle massage with mandarin can help relieve symptoms. Topical applications support healthy, glowing skin; if you would like to reduce the appearance of stretch marks or scars, try remedies that include mandarin.

- Diffuse mandarin alone or with other citrus oils, such as sweet orange and lemon, to reduce stress and create a pleasant, relaxed atmosphere.
- In times of emotional difficulty, add mandarin to an aromatherapy inhaler and breathe deeply to uplift your spirits.
- Try the Lift Me Up Roll-On (see page 128) when you are feeling exhausted.

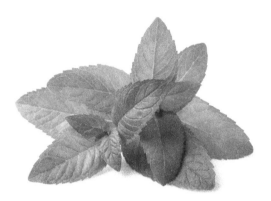

Peppermint
(Mentha piperita)

Peppermint essential oil is cool and refreshing, with a sharp, stimulating scent that enhances focus while increasing mental acuity. It lifts brain fog, increases alertness, and eases depression. Peppermint's ability to alleviate exhaustion and promote stamina while also relieving headaches makes it a valuable ally, particularly on long workdays. This is a great oil to keep in your desk drawer!

SAFETY PRECAUTIONS

Peppermint can irritate sensitive skin and mucous membranes. According to *Essential Oil Safety: A Guide for Health Care Professionals* by Robert Tisserand and Rodney Young, it should not be applied near the faces of infants or children, and it should be avoided by those with G6PD deficiency (a genetic disorder) or cardiac fibrillation (an irregular heartbeat). Peppermint should not be used during pregnancy. If you are nursing, frequent exposure to peppermint can reduce lactation.

SUBSTITUTES

Spearmint

BLENDS WELL WITH

Roman chamomile, rosemary, lemongrass, grapefruit, lime, eucalyptus

HEALING PROPERTIES

1. Decongestant, thins mucus
2. Helps control infection
3. Helps prevent cramping and muscle spasms
4. Reduces fever
5. Reduces gas
6. Relieves pain and offers a numbing effect
7. Stimulates or promotes menstruation
8. Stimulating and uplifting

USES

When properly diluted, peppermint essential oil can be applied topically to relieve rashes, skin irritation, and inflammation. It relieves the pain of a sunburn while offering cool comfort. In stronger concentrations, peppermint penetrates the skin to relieve joint and muscle aches. Inhaled, it is helpful for alleviating cold and flu symptoms. If you have overindulged and are suffering from indigestion, a soothing tummy massage with peppermint can help.

- Diffuse peppermint to help with cold symptoms, headaches, or nausea.
- Prone to travel sickness and do not have an aromatherapy inhaler on hand? Add a few drops of peppermint essential oil to a tissue or cotton pad, seal it inside a small container, and inhale the aroma to banish nausea.
- Try the Refresh My Memory Diffuser Blend (see page 146) if you are feeling a bit foggy.

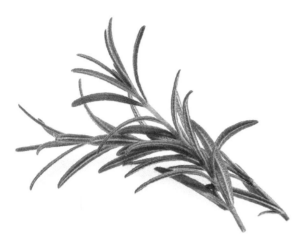

Rosemary
(Rosmarinus officinalis)

The intriguing, herbal scent of rosemary essential oil is clean and crisp with a distinct note of camphor. This invigorating essential oil stimulates the nervous system, which aids focus and promotes an alert, centered feeling. If you are facing a long work or study session or are looking for an alternative to caffeine during a long-distance drive, rosemary is an excellent choice.

SAFETY PRECAUTIONS

Rosemary essential oil should not be used by people with epilepsy nor by those with high blood pressure. It is not suitable for use during pregnancy.

SUBSTITUTES

Sage, thyme, basil

BLENDS WELL WITH

Thyme, basil, spearmint, bergamot, lime, cypress, cedarwood, balsam fir

HEALING PROPERTIES

1. Antidepressant
2. Astringent
3. Balances the nervous system and eases stress
4. Decongestant
5. Energizing and strengthening
6. Promotes urination
7. Relieves pain
8. Stimulates or promotes menstruation
9. Stimulating and uplifting
10. Supports healthy digestion

USES

When inhaled, rosemary essential oil can help ease congestion, cough, bronchitis, and allergy symptoms. Applied topically, its uses range from cleansing, tightening, and stimulating the skin to relieving cramps, aches, and pains. In haircare products, rosemary stimulates the scalp, promoting a healthy scalp while leaving your locks looking shiny and feeling soft.

- If you are suffering from congestion or sinusitis, try diffusing rosemary nearby.
- Create a deep-conditioning treatment by combining 5 drops rosemary essential oil with 1 tablespoon carrier oil. Apply it to your hair and scalp. Let it sit for at least 5 minutes, and then shampoo and condition as usual.
- Try the Productivity Diffuser Blend (see page 130) when mental fatigue slows you down.

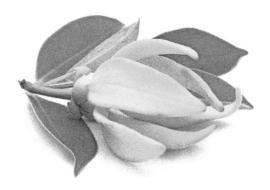

Ylang-ylang
(Cananga odorata)

Offering an intriguing fragrance that incorporates notes of fruity sweetness, ylang-ylang is floral and exotic. This fragrant oil gently eliminates negativity and dispels anger. It comforts in times of bereavement and soothes frayed nerves. If you are feeling overwhelmed, ylang-ylang can help reduce some of the burden and help you find stillness.

SAFETY PRECAUTIONS

High concentrations of ylang-ylang can sometimes cause headaches. *Essential Oil Safety: A Guide for Health Care Professionals* by Robert Tisserand and Rodney Young, cautions against use on diseased, damaged, or highly sensitive skin and on children under the age of two.

SUBSTITUTES

Neroli, rose, jasmine

BLENDS WELL WITH

Bergamot, patchouli, lavender, vetiver, peppermint, orange, cinnamon, clove

HEALING PROPERTIES

1. Aids in sleep and deep relaxation
2. Antianxiety
3. Antibacterial
4. Antidepressant
5. Antiseptic
6. Aphrodisiac
7. Balances the nervous system and eases stress
8. Helps control dry, itchy skin
9. Lowers blood pressure
10. Promotes feelings of happiness

USES

While ylang-ylang is most famous for its usefulness in emotional work, it soothes skin, too. Whether your skin is overly dry or too oily, you can promote balance by adding this elegant essential oil to your skincare routine. Ylang-ylang's antibacterial and antiseptic properties make it a gentle treatment for acne and a comforting, cleansing addition to first-aid treatments.

- Ease tension, anxiety, grief, or shock by diffusing ylang-ylang.
- If you feel panic setting in, try directly inhaling ylang-ylang. It can help bring you back to center while easing physical manifestations of panic, such as rapid breathing.
- Try the In the Mood Linen Spray (see page 168) to boost libido and create a romantic atmosphere in your bedroom.

ESSENTIAL OIL	BLENDS WELL WITH	USES	HEALING PROPERTIES
BALSAM FIR (Abies balsamea)	All citrus oils, bergamot mint, cedarwood, peppermint, pine, spearmint	Anxiety, depression, fatigue, respiratory health, tension	Antiseptic, pain-relieving, refreshing, stimulating, uplifting
BASIL (Ocimum basilicum)	All citrus oils, cedarwood, ginger	Cold and flu, exhaustion, mental drain, lack of motivation	Antidepressant, energizing, focusing
BERGAMOT MINT (Mentha aquatica)	All citrus oils, basil, geranium, lavender	Respiratory health, sadness, stress, tension	Clarifying, harmonizing, refreshing, uplifting
BLUE TANSY (Tanacetum annuum)	Clary sage, geranium, lavender, spearmint, ylang-ylang	Impatience, muscle aches, overthinking	Anti-inflammatory, focusing, relaxing
CEDARWOOD (Cedrus atlantica)	Bergamot, lavender, lemon, Roman chamomile	Conflict, mindfulness, resilience, skin irritation	Antiseptic, calming, grounding, soothing
CINNAMON (Cinnamomum zeylanicum)	All citrus oils, clove, ginger, lemongrass, nutmeg	Cold and flu, emotional distress, indigestion, sore joints and muscles	Energizing, pain-relieving, stimulating, warming
CLOVE (Syzygium aromaticum)	All citrus oils, cinnamon, ginger, nutmeg	Courage, inner strength, mental fog, toothache	Invigorating, pain-relieving, stimulating, warming

ESSENTIAL OIL	BLENDS WELL WITH	USES	HEALING PROPERTIES
CORIANDER (Coriandrum sativum)	All citrus oils, bergamot, cinnamon, ginger, neroli	Aches and pains, fatigue, indigestion, migraine, nausea	Pain-relieving, digestive health, invigorating, stimulating
CYPRESS (Cupressus sempervirens)	Bergamot, clary sage, frankincense, lavender, marjoram, pine, sandalwood	Anger, bloating, feeling overwhelmed, nervousness, skin healing	Balancing, calming, stabilizing, strengthening
EUCALYPTUS (Eucalyptus radiata)	Lavender, lemon, lemongrass, pine, tea tree, thyme	Aches and pains, first aid, focus, low energy, respiratory issues	Decongestant, focusing, pain-relieving, refreshing
FENNEL (Foeniculum vulgare)	Cedarwood, cinnamon, grapefruit, lemon, peppermint, spearmint	Clarity, contentment, digestive health, fluid retention, focus, weight management	Balancing, diuretic, skin tonic, stimulating
GINGER (Zingiber officinale)	All citrus oils, cinnamon, clove, nutmeg	Aches and pains, circulation, low energy, motion sickness, nausea	Aphrodisiac, energizing, uplifting, warming
GRAPEFRUIT (Citrus paradisi)	All citrus oils, all spicy oils, balsam fir, frankincense, pine, spikenard	Bloating, depression, nervousness, sadness, sluggishness, water retention	Diuretic, energizing, euphoric, focusing, grounding

ESSENTIAL OIL	BLENDS WELL WITH	USES	HEALING PROPERTIES
HELICHRYSUM (Helichrysum italicum)	Bergamot, clary sage, lavandin, lavender, mandarin, Roman chamomile, spikenard	Exhaustion, first aid, general skin health, grief, hopelessness, nervousness, skin irritation	Anti-inflammatory, encouraging, pain-relieving, regenerative
HOLY BASIL (Ocimum tenuiflorum)	Bergamot, clary sage, geranium, lavender, lemongrass, rosemary, sweet orange, thyme	Anxiety, cramping and muscle spasms, focus, low energy, nervous tension, respiratory health, stress	Antispasmodic, energizing, grounding, pain-relieving, uplifting
HYSSOP (Hyssopus officinalis)	Clary sage, geranium, lemon, mandarin, melissa, rosemary, sweet orange	Aches and pains, digestive health, emotional trauma, respiratory health, spiritual awareness	Antiseptic, antispasmodic, balancing, encouraging, stimulating
JASMINE (Jasminum grandiflorum)	Frankincense, geranium, lavender, neroli, patchouli, rose, rose geranium, sandalwood	Depression, despondence, fatigue, frustration, insomnia, skin balancing, stress	Aphrodisiac, balancing, comforting, joyful, uplifting
LAVANDIN (Lavandula x intermedia)	Bergamot, cinnamon, clary sage, jasmine, lemongrass, patchouli, pine, rosemary, thyme	Boredom, discomfort, respiratory health, restlessness, tension	Antidepressant, comforting, expectorant, stimulating

ESSENTIAL OIL	BLENDS WELL WITH	USES	HEALING PROPERTIES
LEMONGRASS (Cymbopogon flexuosus)	Basil, cedarwood, geranium, holy basil, jasmine, lavender, tea tree	Clarity, creativity, focus, gastro-intestinal health, inspiration, lethargy	Antibacterial, antidepressant, stimulating
LIME (Citrus × aurantiifolia)	All citrus oils, clary sage, lavandin, lavender, neroli, sage, ylang-ylang	Depression, dull skin, exhaustion, overthinking, respiratory health, withdrawal	Cheerful, energizing, refreshing, restorative
MARJORAM (Origanum majorana)	Clary sage, grapefruit, lavender, rosemary, sage, thyme	Aches and pains, anxiety, digestive health, grief, insomnia, loss, obsessive thought patterns, regret, stress	Balancing, digestive health, expectorant, nurturing, pain-relieving, relaxing
MELISSA (Melissa officinalis)	Basil, geranium, lavender, Roman chamomile, rose, rose geranium, ylang-ylang	Acne, anger, anxiety, depression, oily skin, panic, resentment, stress	Antidepressant, antibacterial, balancing, comforting, relaxing
MYRRH (Commiphora myrrha)	Clove, frankincense, lavender, patchouli, Roman chamomile, sandalwood	Chapped skin, destructive thought patterns, imbalance, meditation, numbness, oral health	Antibacterial, antifungal, detoxifying, harmonizing, peaceful

ESSENTIAL OIL	BLENDS WELL WITH	USES	HEALING PROPERTIES
NEROLI (Citrus × aurantium)	All citrus oils, geranium, jasmine, lavender, rose, rose geranium, sandalwood, ylang-ylang	Cramps and muscle spasms, fear, feeling withdrawn, headaches, sadness, scars and stretch marks, shock, stress, uncertainty	Antispasmodic, balancing, clarifying, pacifying, regenerative, rejuvenating
NUTMEG (Myristica fragrans)	All citrus oils, clary sage, clove, cypress, geranium, ginger, rosemary	Digestive complaints, feeling stuck, focus, motivation, muscle and joint pain	Aphrodisiac, energizing, pain-relieving, stimulating, warming
PATCHOULI (Pogostemon cablin)	Bergamot, clary sage, frankincense, geranium, lavender, myrrh, rose, rose geranium, sandalwood, ylang-ylang	Addiction, anxiety, feelings of emptiness, meditation, sadness, skincare, scars and stretch marks, worry	Antidepressant, astringent, diuretic, freeing, grounding, relaxing
PINE (Pinus sylvestris)	All citrus oils, cedarwood, clary sage, eucalyptus, balsam fir, lavender, rosemary, sage	Fatigue, feeling overwhelmed, focus, mental clarity, muscle and joint pain, negative emotions, respiratory health	Antimicrobial, cleansing, clearing, energizing, uplifting, restorative

ESSENTIAL OIL	BLENDS WELL WITH	USES	HEALING PROPERTIES
ROMAN CHAMOMILE (Chamaemelum nobile)	Bergamot, clary sage, grapefruit, lavender, lemon, rose, rosemary, sage, tea tree, vetiver, ylang-ylang	Anger, depression, fear, headaches, impatience, insomnia, irritability, loneliness, panic, restlessness, skincare, stress	Anti-inflammatory, calming, nourishing, relaxing, soothing
ROSE (Rosa damascena)	Bergamot, clary sage, clove, fennel, geranium, ginger, jasmine, neroli, Roman chamomile, rose geranium, sandalwood, vetiver	Anger, depression, grief, menopause, menstrual issues, nervousness, PTSD, self-esteem, shock, skincare, stress, trauma	Antidepressant, harmonizing, healing, nurturing, promotes forgiveness, relaxing
ROSE GERANIUM (Pelargonium capitatum)	All citrus oils, basil, bergamot, cedarwood, clary sage, lemongrass, neroli	Anxiety, bloating, depression, menopause, PMS, skincare, stress, tension	Antianxiety, antidepressant, balancing, detoxifying, diuretic, energizing
SAGE (Salvia officinalis)	Bergamot, lavandin, lavender, lemon, lime, peppermint, rosemary, spearmint	Digestive health, emotional upset, grief, headaches, muscle and joint pain, memory, mental fatigue, nervousness, sore throat	Antibacterial, anti-inflammatory, balancing, diuretic, pain-relieving, relaxing

ESSENTIAL OIL	BLENDS WELL WITH	USES	HEALING PROPERTIES
SANDALWOOD (Santalum album)	Bergamot, geranium, lavender, myrrh, rose, spikenard, vetiver, ylang-ylang	Depression, meditation, pressure, self-doubt, scars and stretch marks, skincare, stress	Aphrodisiac, balancing, calming, grounding, pacifying, unifying
SPEARMINT (Mentha spicata)	Basil, eucalyptus, holy basil, lavender, rosemary, tea tree	Digestive health, headaches and migraines, mental fatigue, nausea, nervousness, oral health, respiratory health	Decongestant, digestive, playful, refreshing, restorative, stimulating
SPIKENARD (Nardostachys jatamansi)	Clary sage, frankincense, lemon, myrrh, neroli, patchouli, vetiver	Anger, emotional upset, exhaustion, insomnia, meditation, migraine, tension, worry	Balancing, calming, grounding, relaxing, restorative
SWEET ORANGE (Citrus × aurantium)	All citrus oils, cinnamon, clove, frankincense, ginger, myrrh, nutmeg, sandalwood, vetiver	Anxiety, cold and flu, digestive health, nervous tension, oral health, sadness, skin balancing, stress, worry	Antidepressant, antiseptic, diuretic, harmonizing, uplifting
TEA TREE (Melaleuca alternifolia)	Cinnamon, clary sage, clove, eucalyptus, lavandin, lavender, lemon, peppermint, rosemary, thyme	Aches and pains, acne, athlete's foot, cold and flu, exhaustion, first aid, haircare, headache, shock, sinusitis, skincare	Antibacterial, antifungal, antiseptic, refreshing, stimulating

ESSENTIAL OIL	BLENDS WELL WITH	USES	HEALING PROPERTIES
THYME (Thymus vulgaris)	Basil, bergamot, balsam fir, holy basil, lavandin, lavender, pine, rosemary, sage	Aches and pains, cold and flu, concentration, fear, memory, nervousness, respiratory health	Antibacterial, expectorant, pain-relieving, stimulating
VALERIAN (Valeriana officinalis)	Clary sage, lavandin, lavender, marjoram, Roman chamomile	Anxiety, cramps and muscle spasms, gastrointestinal health, insomnia, nervousness, skincare	Balancing, calming, comforting, relaxing
VETIVER (Chrysopogon zizanioides)	All citrus oils, frankincense, jasmine, lavender, Roman chamomile, sandalwood, ylang-ylang	Aches and pains, anger, burnout, grief, insomnia, irritation, meditation, restlessness, stress, skincare, tension	Balancing, focusing, reassuring, relaxing, soothing, stabilizing
YARROW (Achillea millefolium)	Clary sage, eucalyptus, geranium, lavender, peppermint, sage, spearmint	Aches and pains, anger, first aid, meditation, self-awareness, trauma	Anti-inflammatory, antiseptic, balancing, refreshing, stabilizing

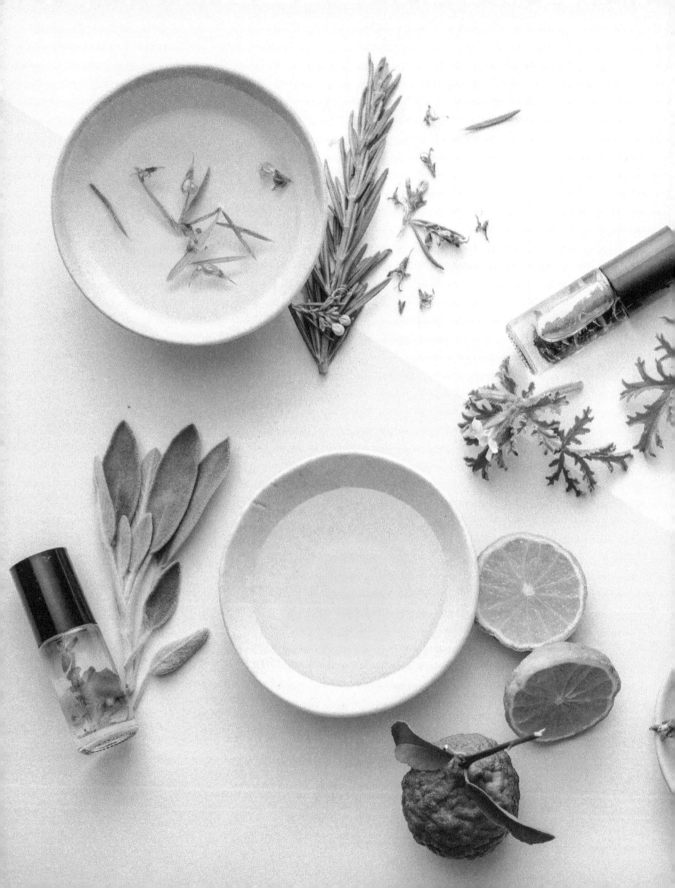

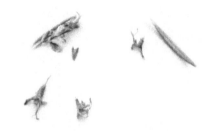

PART TWO

Aromatherapy Remedies *for* Self-Care

Now that you have gotten to know some of the top essential oils a little better, it is time to start combining them to help address your self-care needs. In this part, you will find remedy blends for your emotional, mental, and physical needs, organized by symptom. I have also included several self-care-boost tips along the way— try to include these whenever possible to reach your goals faster.

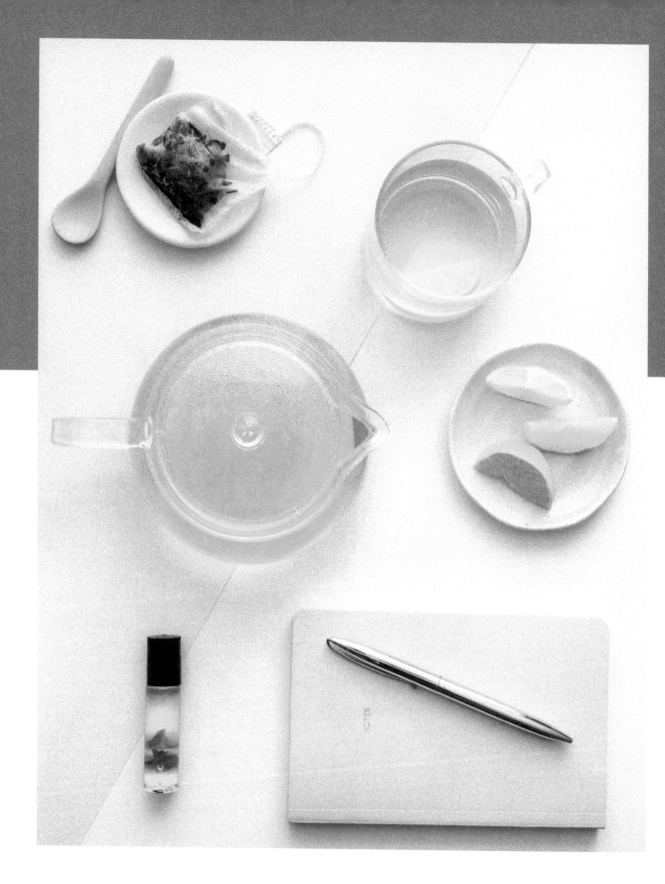

05

Emotional Well-Being

Whether you are looking for a way to improve your mood or deal with tough emotions like anger, fear, or frustration, you'll find a blend in this chapter that will fit the bill. Soothing essential oils like lavender, Roman chamomile, and blue tansy are great for helping you cope when stress and anxiety are interfering with your life, while energizing favorites like lemon, bergamot, and grapefruit can help you chase away the blues with their uplifting benefits.

Remember that although aromatherapy is a great way to practice self-care, other self-care steps are also essential—whether it's carving out time for your own emotional needs, seeking therapy, evaluating your relationships, or making additional lifestyle changes. So, enjoy these remedies, seek a supportive environment, and work toward a healthy lifestyle overall. You will emerge happier, more resilient, and more energetic.

ANGER RELEASE DIFFUSER BLEND

This soothing blend calms the intense heat of anger with lavender and ylang-ylang to relax the mind and Roman chamomile helps restore balance. If you are emotionally overloaded and need to distance yourself from a negative situation, this simple diffusion can help.

DIFFUSION, SAFE FOR AGES 2+, DO NOT USE IF PREGNANT

3 drops Roman chamomile essential oil

2 drops lavender essential oil

2 drops ylang-ylang essential oil

1. Add the essential oils directly to your diffuser, following the manufacturer's instructions.

2. While the diffuser is running, breathe deeply and remind yourself that anger is a normal and valid emotion. Try to find its root cause; fear, pain, and frustration are common ones. The goal is not to get stuck in anger, so focus on finding an actionable step to deal with the cause, which will allow you to move forward.

SELF-CARE BOOST: Breathing through anger can help. Focus on your breath, counting to 5 on each inhalation, holding your breath for 5 seconds, and counting to 5 on each exhalation. Try to let go of the anger, recognizing that holding on to it harms you but releasing it frees you from the uncomfortable sensation. As you continue this work, try extending your exhalations until they are a few seconds longer than each inhalation. This tells your brain that you are in a restful state and out of danger.

ANTIANXIETY INHALER

With peaceful jasmine, uplifting lemon, and tranquil vetiver, this synergistic blend reduces anxiety by allowing your mind to relax and come to center so you can purge thoughts that are not helping now and focus on what is important. If you finvd yourself ruminating, reach for this inhaler to interrupt looping thoughts and reduce the tension that accompanies anxiety. **DIRECT INHALATION, SAFE FOR AGES 2+**

9 drops jasmine
  essential oil
6 drops lemon essential oil
1 drop vetiver essential oil

1. Put the essential oils in a small glass or ceramic bowl. Swirl the bowl around to blend the oils.

2. Put the cotton wick from the aromatherapy inhaler in the bowl and allow the wick to absorb the blend.

3. With a pair of tweezers, place the saturated wick into the aromatherapy inhaler and assemble. Snap or screw the cap into place. Affix a label to the inhaler.

4. Open the cap and inhale deeply through your nose to reduce anxiety as often as needed.

ACUPRESSURE TIP: The acupressure point Pericardium 6 (located the width of 3 fingers below the center of your inner wrist crease) is a great point to help settle the mind. Dilute 1 drop vetiver or jasmine with 1 teaspoon carrier oil and massage the blend on this point for 90 seconds to reduce anxiety.

ANXIETY BEGONE DIFFUSER BLEND

With refreshing bergamot and soothing lavender, this simple diffuser blend calms racing thoughts while encouraging gentle relaxation. In studies, this blend has been shown to help anxiety, stress, and depression. When negative thoughts, worries, and fears race through your head, lavender and bergamot can help you begin the process of restoring balance.

DIFFUSION, SAFE FOR AGES 2+

5 drops lavender essential oil

5 drops bergamot essential oil

1. Add the essential oils directly to your diffuser, following the manufacturer's instructions.

2. While the diffuser is running, relax and inhale.

DIRECT INHALATION OPTION: For direct inhalation of this calming blend, use equal drops of lavender and bergamot to saturate the wick of an aromatherapy inhaler. (See the Antianxiety Inhaler on page 79 for instructions.)

SELF-CARE BOOST: When we drink coffee and other beverages that contain caffeine, the activity in our autonomic nervous system increases, which can kick in the fight-or-flight response. So, if anxiety intrudes often, consider cutting back on the caffeine.

UPLIFTING DIFFUSER BLEND

Since depression can cause physical symptoms as well as emotional ones, this diffuser blend relies on essential oils that help relieve anxiety, sadness, difficulty concentrating, and stress. Both uplifting and relaxing, this blend can make it easier to manage your feelings and improve your mood while easing the apprehension that often accompanies depression.

DIFFUSION, SAFE FOR AGES 2+, DO NOT USE IF PREGNANT

10 drops bergamot essential oil

10 drops lavender essential oil

10 drops lemon essential oil

10 drops peppermint essential oil

10 drops sweet orange essential oil

10 drops ylang-ylang essential oil

5 drops patchouli essential oil

1. Put all of the essential oils in a small, dark-colored bottle. (If you are using a pipette to measure out the oils, use a new one for each essential oil—do not reuse.)

2. Cap the bottle tightly and swirl to blend the oils.

3. Add 8 to 10 drops of the blend to your diffuser, following the manufacturer's instructions. Label and store the remaining blend.

4. While the diffuser is running, simply relax and breathe or practice a mindfulness meditation for 10 to 15 minutes while enjoying the beautiful aroma.

SELF-CARE BOOST: Aromatherapy can be a wonderful complement to conventional treatments for depression. However, if you take prescription antidepressants, speak to your health-care practitioner for guidance and advice on how best to use essential oils alongside your medication before getting started.

JOYFUL SPIRIT INHALER

Elevate your mood quickly with this delightful blend. Studies show that the aromatic molecules in essential oils have the ability to cross the blood-brain barrier and positively impact the limbic system, controlling feelings of depression as well as the stress and anxiety that often come with it. Together, jasmine, clary sage, and rose calm anxiety and encourage a hopeful outlook. Reach for this inhaler when you first notice that you are feeling low.

DIRECT INHALATION, SAFE FOR AGES 6+, DO NOT USE IF PREGNANT

8 drops jasmine
   essential oil
6 drops rose
   essential oil (optional)
4 drops clary sage
   essential oil

1. Put the essential oils in a small glass or ceramic bowl. Swirl the bowl around to blend the oils.

2. Put the cotton wick from the aromatherapy inhaler in the bowl and allow the wick to absorb the blend.

3. With a pair of tweezers, place the saturated wick into the aromatherapy inhaler and assemble. Snap or screw the cap into place. Affix a label to the inhaler.

4. Open the cap and inhale deeply through your nose to lift your spirits as often as needed.

SELF-CARE BOOST: Change your food, change your mood! New research is showing how important diet is for regulating our overall mood. Eating foods that keep blood sugar levels stable (such as unrefined "slow" carbs) and getting plenty of micronutrient-rich fruits and vegetables (which help create feel-good chemicals in the brain) are vital to emotional well-being.

COURAGEOUS HEART INHALER

Fear is meant to keep us safe, but too often, it stops us from stepping forward and taking action to live our best lives. Calming lavender, grounding vetiver, reassuring bergamot, and comforting cedarwood can help redirect your focus when chaotic thoughts and hectic situations threaten to damage your resolve. Reach for this inhaler anytime you require a touch of courage to move forward. **DIRECT INHALATION, SAFE FOR AGES 6+**

---

5 drops lavender essential oil

4 drops cedarwood essential oil

4 drops vetiver essential oil

3 drops bergamot essential oil

1. Put the essential oils in a small glass or ceramic bowl. Swirl the bowl around to blend the oils.

2. Put the cotton wick from the aromatherapy inhaler in the bowl and allow the wick to absorb the blend.

3. With a pair of tweezers, place the saturated wick into the aromatherapy inhaler and assemble. Snap or screw the cap into place. Affix a label to the inhaler.

4. Open the cap and inhale deeply through your nose to ease your fear as often as needed.

ACUPRESSURE TIP: If your chest tightens when fear strikes, try this: Ren 17, which is located in the center of the sternum, is a great point to help open the chest and get stuck energy moving again. Apply 1 drop bergamot essential oil diluted with 1 teaspoon carrier oil to this point and massage in circular motion for up to 90 seconds. You will be able to take a deep breath again in no time!

SELF-CARE BOOST: If you are often fearful, consider learning more about a tool called emotional freedom technique (EFT). In EFT, you gently tap on the meridian points on your body to reduce a negative emotion—in this case, fear. This method works pretty quickly, and with consistent use over time it can even alleviate specific fears for good.

TRIUMPH DIFFUSER BLEND

This simple, delightful blend can replace exasperation with an immediate sense of satisfaction, flipping your internal switch from a place of irritation and annoyance to one of pleased fulfillment. Patchouli is a great oil for grounding and sweet orange can lift your spirits. Together, these oils create a sweet scent that can snap you out of your frustration funk.

DIFFUSION, SAFE FOR AGES 2+

6 drops sweet orange
 essential oil
4 drops patchouli
 essential oil

1. Add the essential oils directly to your diffuser, following the manufacturer's instructions.

2. While the diffuser is running, practice deep breathing to put the part of your brain that deals with higher reasoning back in control; this will help you rationally work through your thoughts and come to terms with the source of your frustration.

DIRECT INHALATION OPTION: To combat frustration on the go, saturate the wick of an aromatherapy inhaler with this blend, increasing the drops as needed while maintaining the 3:2 ratio between sweet orange and patchouli. (See Antianxiety Inhaler on page 79 for instructions.) Breathe deeply from your inhaler when you are stuck in traffic, waiting in line, or dealing with other frustrating scenarios.

SELF-CARE BOOST: If you often find yourself feeling frustrated, spend some time thinking about what tends to trigger your feelings of irritation. When you are aware of your triggers and the thoughts that arise in response to them, you can take steps to avoid the triggers or make a conscious effort to change how you respond.

CHEERFUL DIFFUSER BLEND

This warm, inviting blend is the ideal antidote to gloomy weather and dark moods. With uplifting sweet orange, supportive nutmeg, energizing cinnamon, and intriguing clove, it balances emotions and brightens your spirits. **DIFFUSION, SAFE FOR AGES 2+, DO NOT USE IF PREGNANT OR BREASTFEEDING**

30 drops sweet orange essential oil
20 drops cinnamon essential oil
10 drops clove essential oil
10 drops nutmeg essential oil

1. Put each of the essential oils in a small, dark-colored bottle. (If you are using a pipette to measure out the oils, use a new one for each essential oil—do not reuse.)
2. Cap the bottle tightly and swirl to blend the oils.
3. Add 8 to 10 drops of the blend to your diffuser, following the manufacturer's instructions. Label and store the remaining blend.
4. While the diffuser is running, enjoy the uplifting aroma as you go about your usual activities.

SELF-CARE BOOST: To snap yourself out of a gloomy mood, shake up your routine by doing something fun while your diffuser is running. Here are a few ideas: Work on a creative project, have a private dance party in your kitchen, or reach out to a friend who makes you laugh.

EMOTIONAL HEALING INHALER

Shock, anger, numbness, and guilt are just a few of the emotions we encounter when we grieve. Aromatherapy does not erase the pain of loss, but it can help you cope by allowing your mind to relax, focus on the present, slow down, and work through this complicated emotion. With rose to soothe the sensation of loss, orange to gently lift you up, and vetiver to calm and ground you, this blend can make it easier to get through difficult days. **DIRECT INHALATION, SAFE FOR AGES 6+**

6 drops sweet orange
  essential oil
2 drops rose essential oil
2 drops vetiver essential oil

1. Put the essential oils in a small glass or ceramic bowl. Swirl the bowl around to blend the oils.

2. Put the cotton wick from the aromatherapy inhaler in the bowl and allow the wick to absorb the blend.

3. With a pair of tweezers, place the saturated wick into the aromatherapy inhaler and assemble. Snap or screw the cap into place. Affix a label to the inhaler.

4. Open the cap and inhale deeply through your nose as often as needed.

SELF-CARE BOOST: Grief is exhausting and it can take a toll on your entire body. During this time, do what you can to care for your physical health: Stay hydrated, eat well, get plenty of fresh air, and moisturize your skin. Take whatever responsibilities you can off your plate and allow yourself plenty of downtime.

KEEP MOVING FORWARD DIFFUSER BLEND

Sadness may be causing you to feel stuck and unmotivated, but this blend can help you heal and move forward. Frankincense slows racing thoughts and promotes a sense of calm, while neroli soothes your senses and combats the feelings of anxiety, stress, and depression that often accompany loss. Use this blend anytime you begin to feel as if you cannot take another step. **DIFFUSION, SAFE FOR AGES 6+**

20 drops neroli essential oil
20 drops frankincense
essential oil

1. Put the essential oils in a small, dark-colored bottle. (If you are using a pipette to measure out the oils, use a new one for each essential oil—do not reuse.)

2. Cap the bottle tightly and swirl to blend the oils.

3. Add 8 to 10 drops of the blend to your diffuser, following the manufacturer's instructions. Label and store the remaining blend.

4. While the diffuser is running, sit back and allow the feelings of being stuck and unmotivated to fade.

DIRECT INHALATION OPTION: If you would like to use this on the go, use 8 to 10 drops of this blend in an aromatherapy inhaler. (See Antianxiety Inhaler on page 79 for instructions.) Breathe deeply from your inhaler as often as needed to keep yourself moving forward.

HOPEFUL OUTLOOK ROLL-ON

Sometimes life's challenges drag us down, making it difficult to see or imagine brighter days ahead. With calming, supportive lavandin, cheerful grapefruit, and invigorating geranium, this encouraging roll-on can help you find inner strength and foster a hopeful outlook.

TOPICAL, SAFE FOR AGES 6+

3 drops grapefruit essential oil

2 drops geranium essential oil

1 drop lavandin essential oil

1¾ teaspoons jojoba oil

1. Using a fresh pipette for each oil, put the essential oils in a prelabeled 10-milliliter roller bottle. Add the jojoba oil.

2. Snap on the rollerball and screw on the cap. Shake until well-mixed.

3. Roll onto your wrists and other pulse points as needed for a change in perspective.

SELF-CARE BOOST: Go outside for a little bit of fresh air and sunshine. Breathing in fresh air and feeling sunshine on your skin can improve your outlook in a matter of minutes.

MY "I'VE GOT THIS" INHALER

When you are overcome with worry about what others think, this blend can help bring you back to a place of self-acceptance. With joyful hints of lemon and lime, grounding patchouli, and comforting cedarwood, it slows down those anxious thoughts and helps you replace them with more positive emotions. Whether insecurity is a constant companion or if you are concerned about something specific, this inhaler can help you create a more positive reality. **DIRECT INHALATION, SAFE FOR AGES 6+**

4 drops lemon essential oil

2 drops cedarwood essential oil

2 drops lime essential oil

1 drop patchouli essential oil

1. Put the essential oils in a small glass or ceramic bowl. Swirl the bowl around to blend the oils.

2. Put the cotton wick from the aromatherapy inhaler in the bowl and allow the wick to absorb the blend.

3. With a pair of tweezers, place the saturated wick into the aromatherapy inhaler and assemble. Snap or screw the cap into place. Affix a label to the inhaler.

4. Open the cap and inhale deeply through your nose as often as needed to remind yourself that you have got this!

SELF-CARE BOOST: Forgive yourself for slip-ups, and do not be too demanding with yourself. Giving yourself a hard time is harmful and counterproductive. Check in on your self-talk. If you are saying things to yourself that you would not say to a friend or loved one, take time to rewrite your script, making it kind and motivational.

GOODBYE GRUMPINESS INHALER

When you are feeling overwhelmed and stressed, irritability can make matters worse. This refreshing blend helps you gather your thoughts, relax your mind, and take the pressure off. Uplifting balsam fir and joyful bergamot activate your brain's pleasure center, whereas crisp basil offers a calming, stabilizing presence. When emotional tension surfaces, this inhaler can help you restore balance. **DIRECT INHALATION, SAFE FOR AGES 6+**

6 drops balsam fir
  essential oil
2 drops bergamot
  essential oil
1 drop basil essential oil

1. Put the essential oils in a small glass or ceramic bowl. Swirl the bowl around to blend the oils.

2. Put the cotton wick from the aromatherapy inhaler into the bowl and allow the wick to absorb the blend.

3. With a pair of tweezers, place the saturated wick into the aromatherapy inhaler and assemble. Snap or screw the cap into place. Affix a label to the inhaler.

4. Open the cap and inhale deeply through your nose as often as needed to ward away grumpiness.

SELF-CARE BOOST: After using this inhaler, ask yourself what is causing your irritability. You may discover that it is something as simple as being hungry or overtired. If so, be sure to tend to your basic needs: Have a healthy snack to tide you over if you need one or take a power nap if there is a place and time for it.

IRRITABILITY BEGONE DIFFUSER BLEND

Irritability can be a messy mix of anger, agitation, and frustration—usually brought on by stress, overwhelming anxiety, sleep deprivation, and more. This blend targets the physical and psychological factors with irresistibly cheerful mandarin, buoyant grapefruit, and spicy, grounding clove. Diffused in your home, it can help you restore positive feelings and power throughout the rest of your day. **DIFFUSION, SAFE FOR AGES 2+, DO NOT USE IF PREGNANT**

10 drops clove essential oil

10 drops grapefruit essential oil

10 drops mandarin essential oil

1. Put the essential oils in a small, dark-colored bottle. (If you are using a pipette to measure out the oils, use a new one for each essential oil—do not reuse.)

2. Cap the bottle tightly and swirl to blend the oils.

3. Add 8 to 10 drops of the blend to your diffuser, following the manufacturer's instructions. Label and store the remaining blend.

4. While the diffuser is running, enjoy the scent of cheeriness permeating your space.

DIRECT INHALATION OPTION: If you would like to use this remedy on the go, use 8 to 10 drops of this blend in an aromatherapy inhaler. (See Antianxiety Inhaler on page 79 for instructions.) Breathe deeply from your inhaler as often as needed to turn your frown upside down.

ACUPRESSURE TIP: In Traditional Chinese Medicine, irritability is often a sign of liver qi stagnation—that is, stuck energy in your liver meridian. To get your qi moving properly again, massage the following points with diluted mandarin essential oil: Liver 3 (located between the webbing of your first and second toes, about 1 inch toward the ankle) and Large Intestine 4 (located on the backside of the hand, on the fleshy mound between the thumb and index finger). Massage each point for up to 90 seconds, alternating sides.

LOVE MYSELF INHALER

This uplifting blend treats you to an indulgent, enticing fragrance that allows your mind to focus on the good things. Bergamot mint (which differs from regular bergamot) inspires creativity and encourages you to seek enjoyment, whereas bergamot, sage, and marjoram add rich, grounding warmth. Lavender's presence is soothing and relaxing, encouraging you to find pleasure in your own company. **DIRECT INHALATION, SAFE FOR AGES 6+, DO NOT USE IF PREGNANT OR BREASTFEEDING**

3 drops bergamot mint essential oil

3 drops lavender essential oil

2 drops bergamot essential oil

1 drop marjoram essential oil

1 drop sage essential oil

1. Put the essential oils in a small glass or ceramic bowl. Swirl the bowl around to blend the oils.

2. Put the cotton wick from the aromatherapy inhaler in the bowl and allow the wick to absorb the blend.

3. With a pair of tweezers, place the saturated wick into the aromatherapy inhaler and assemble. Snap or screw the cap into place. Affix a label to the inhaler.

4. Open the cap and inhale deeply through your nose as often as needed.

SELF-CARE BOOST: Remind yourself that your "me time" is precious. When you make time to care for yourself, your body thanks you—and you can thank your body for being there for you, too. Think of a few things you are grateful for when it comes to your body. It could be a simple compliment or something more general like being grateful for your strong legs, which hold you up every day. Practicing gratitude is a great way to notice all the wonderful things in your life, including you.

CHEER UP DIFFUSER BLEND

With bright notes of bergamot and sweet orange, plus comforting hints of rose and geranium, this warm, summery fragrance eases all types of melancholy. If your thoughts are a bit cluttered, the citrus oils will help you focus. Mingled with lightly sweet florals, they will also help stop the downward spiral of negativity. **DIFFUSION, SAFE FOR AGES 2+**

15 drops bergamot
essential oil
10 drops geranium
essential oil
5 drops sweet orange
essential oil
5 drops rose essential oil

1. Put the essential oils in a small, dark-colored bottle. (If you are using a pipette to measure out the oils, use a new one for each essential oil—do not reuse.)
2. Cap the bottle tightly and swirl to blend the oils.
3. Add 8 to 10 drops of the blend to your diffuser, following the manufacturer's instructions. Label and store the remaining blend.
4. While the diffuser is running, feel the melancholy floating away.

SELF-CARE BOOST: Feeling bored or a little down? Do something creative to focus your mind on something other than what's got you out of sorts. Make it something you already enjoy that is simple and fun. Adult coloring books and puzzles, for example, put your brain to work without asking too much of you.

SUNNY OUTLOOK INHALER

This cheerful blend alleviates feelings of melancholy, allowing the mind to release that sense of sadness that is lurking just beneath the surface. Sweet orange, lime, and grapefruit are cheerful reminders of good times to come and together their crisp fragrance lifts the mental fog that often accompanies melancholy. Reach for this inhaler anytime you would like to embrace a happier mood. **DIRECT INHALATION, SAFE FOR AGES 6+**

5 drops grapefruit
essential oil

5 drops sweet orange
essential oil

2 drops lime essential oil

1. Put the essential oils in a small glass or ceramic bowl. Swirl the bowl around to blend the oils.

2. Put the cotton wick from the aromatherapy inhaler in the bowl and allow the wick to absorb the blend.

3. With a pair of tweezers, place the saturated wick into the aromatherapy inhaler and assemble. Snap or screw the cap into place. Affix a label to the inhaler.

4. Open the cap and inhale deeply through your nose as often as needed for a sunnier outlook.

ACUPRESSURE TIP: If you are feeling down, try this: Trace a line from the highest point of your ear to the top of your head. You have landed on the point DU 20. To quickly lift your spirits, massage 1 drop grapefruit essential oil diluted with 1 teaspoon carrier oil on this point for up to 90 seconds.

INSTANT MOOD BOOST INHALER

Grounding cedarwood, soothing Roman chamomile, and uplifting sweet orange come together in this lightly spicy, wonderfully balancing blend. Whenever you are feeling moody and mentally overburdened, target tension, irritability, and fatigue with this balancing blend.

DIRECT INHALATION, SAFE FOR AGES 6+, DO NOT USE IF PREGNANT

8 drops cedarwood essential oil

3 drops sweet orange essential oil

2 drops Roman chamomile essential oil

1. Put the essential oils in a small glass or ceramic bowl. Swirl the bowl around to blend the oils.

2. Put the cotton wick from the aromatherapy inhaler in the bowl and allow the wick to absorb the blend.

3. With a pair of tweezers, place the saturated wick into the aromatherapy inhaler and assemble. Snap or screw the cap into place. Affix a label to the inhaler.

4. Open the cap and inhale deeply through your nose to improve your mood as often as needed.

SELF-CARE BOOST: If you are feeling fragile, take some time out for yourself. Try relaxing in a warm bath with 3 drops lavender essential oil blended with 1 teaspoon carrier oil and ½ cup Epsom salts.

BALANCED MOOD DIFFUSER BLEND

When mood swings threaten to disrupt your day, this synergistic blend blows in like a fresh breeze, lifting you up and heightening your spirits. Clean, refreshing eucalyptus adds a touch of depth to invigorating lime and buoyant mandarin, bringing your thoughts back into focus and helping you see the bright side. **DIFFUSION, SAFE FOR AGES 2+**

24 drops lime essential oil
16 drops eucalyptus
  essential oil
16 drops mandarin
  essential oil

1. Put the essential oils in a small, dark-colored bottle. (If you are using a pipette to measure out the oils, use a new one for each essential oil—do not reuse.)

2. Cap the bottle tightly and swirl to blend the oils.

3. Add 8 to 10 drops of the blend to your diffuser, following the manufacturer's instructions. Label and store the remaining blend.

4. While the diffuser is running, sit back and feel yourself coming back into balance.

DIRECT INHALATION OPTION: If you would like to use this remedy on the go, use 8 to 10 drops of this blend in an aromatherapy inhaler. (See Antianxiety Inhaler on page 79 for instructions.) Breathe deeply from your inhaler as often as needed to combat moodiness throughout the day.

THINK POSITIVELY INHALER

This fresh-smelling blend can lift the clouds of negativity in an instant! Crisp, intriguing bergamot and tangy sweet orange provide a touch of citrusy sweetness, contrasting with the warm, mellow notes of clary sage. Melissa is optional, but you can add a drop or two if you have it; it makes this blend even more uplifting. **DIRECT INHALATION, SAFE FOR AGES 6+, DO NOT USE IF PREGNANT OR BREASTFEEDING**

4 drops bergamot
essential oil

2 drops clary sage
essential oil

2 drops melissa essential oil
(optional)

2 drops sweet orange
essential oil

1. Put the essential oils in a small glass or ceramic bowl. Swirl the bowl around to blend the oils.

2. Put the cotton wick from the aromatherapy inhaler in the bowl and allow the wick to absorb the blend.

3. With a pair of tweezers, place the saturated wick into the aromatherapy inhaler and assemble. Snap or screw the cap into place. Affix a label to the inhaler.

4. Open the cap and inhale deeply through your nose as often as needed.

SELF-CARE BOOST: If negativity is weighing on you, try turning it on its head with yoga. Yoga inversions (poses where the legs are in the air) are amazing for quickly changing your mood. For example, the legs-up-the-wall pose is a great one for settling your nervous system and giving you a positivity boost.

CONFIDENCE ROLL-ON

With lavandin for a grounding, calming effect plus refreshing spearmint, this roll-on can help you focus on reality, deal with the task at hand, and eliminate the pent-up stress that typically goes hand in hand with nervousness. The lemon in this blend can help you cope by lowering stress hormones while giving your spirits a welcome lift. **TOPICAL, SAFE FOR AGES 6+**

---

5 drops lavandin
  essential oil
3 drops lemon essential oil
3 drops spearmint
  essential oil
1¾ teaspoons jojoba oil

1. Using a fresh pipette for each oil, place the essential oils in a prelabeled 10-milliliter roller bottle. Add the jojoba oil.

2. Snap on the rollerball and screw on the cap. Shake until well-mixed.

3. Roll onto your wrists and other pulse points as needed.

SELF-CARE BOOST: Got nervous energy? Shake it off! Play your favorite music, turn up the volume, and dance it out. Dancing is an excellent way to dispel some of that nervous energy—and it is fun, too!

CALM AND CLEAR INHALER

Fresh-scented eucalyptus, soothing lavender, and grounding ylang-ylang come together to take your mind off thoughts that lead to nervous tension. Find your center and move forward with a calm sense of purpose with this aromatherapy inhaler. **DIRECT INHALATION, SAFE FOR AGES 6+, DO NOT USE IF PREGNANT**

6 drops eucalyptus
  essential oil
6 drops lavender
  essential oil
4 drops ylang-ylang
  essential oil

1. Put the essential oils in a small glass or ceramic bowl. Swirl the bowl around to blend the oils.

2. Place the cotton wick from the aromatherapy inhaler in the bowl and allow the wick to absorb the blend.

3. With a pair of tweezers, place the saturated wick into the aromatherapy inhaler and assemble. Snap or screw the cap into place. Affix a label to the inhaler.

4. Open the cap and inhale deeply through your nose as often as needed.

SELF-CARE BOOST: Set realistic goals for yourself. Challenges are wonderful and it feels great to reach new heights, but unattainable goals and unrealistic expectations set you up for failure and lead to anxiety, nervous tension, and overwhelm. Set smaller goals and increase the distance as you go.

STOP OVERTHINKING DIFFUSER BLEND

This synergistic blend makes the most of holy basil, which can help you focus when situational anxiety leads to negative thought patterns. Lemon lifts your senses, whereas rosemary sharpens concentration, helps stop the chatter, and places your thoughts on a positive, orderly track. **DIFFUSION, SAFE FOR AGES 2+**

---

24 drops lemon essential oil

16 drops holy basil
essential oil

16 drops rosemary
essential oil

1. Put the essential oils in a small, dark-colored bottle. (If you are using a pipette to measure out the oils, use a new one for each essential oil—do not reuse.)

2. Cap the bottle tightly and swirl to blend the oils.

3. Add 8 to 10 drops of the blend to your diffuser, following the manufacturer's instructions. Label and store the remaining blend.

4. While the diffuser is running, sit back and let your mind take a rest.

DIRECT INHALATION OPTION: If you would like to use this remedy on the go, use 8 to 10 drops of this blend in an aromatherapy inhaler. (See Antianxiety Inhaler on page 79 for instructions.) Breathe deeply from your inhaler as often as needed to keep your thoughts on track throughout the day.

SELF-CARE BOOST: Overthinking can be paralyzing; fortunately, practicing mindfulness can help. A consistent mindfulness practice takes time to cultivate, but it will help you deal with overthinking and other negative thought patterns. Consider downloading a mindfulness app for your smartphone and setting aside time daily to practice.

RESTORE BALANCE DIFFUSER BLEND

This simple, grounding blend brings the warmth and comfort of nutmeg together with the uplifting scent of grapefruit to address the stress and anxiety that tend to lie at the root of overwhelm. Grapefruit enhances focus, too, helping you take a more analytical stance and weigh your options before moving forward. **DIFFUSION, SAFE FOR AGES 2+, DO NOT USE IF PREGNANT OR BREASTFEEDING**

8 drops grapefruit
   essential oil
1 drop nutmeg essential oil

1. Add the essential oils directly to your diffuser, following the manufacturer's instructions.

2. While the diffuser is running, breathe deeply. Focus on each breath, counting to 5 on each inhalation, holding your breath for 5 seconds, and counting to 5 with each exhalation. Focus only on your breath, acknowledging any intruding thoughts and again returning to your breath until your mind feels more relaxed.

3. Once you feel more grounded, organize your thoughts and plan a way to move forward.

STOP STRESSING INHALER

This blend gently redirects your mind, relieving tension and comforting your spirit. Frankincense brings exotic warmth to a refreshing blend of sweet orange and balsam fir, slowing you down and putting you in touch with nature for a moment. When you feel overwhelmed and need to put yourself back on course, reach for this delightful inhaler to reduce the mental strain of stress and anxiety. **DIRECT INHALATION, SAFE FOR AGES 6+**

---

5 drops frankincense
essential oil

3 drops balsam fir
essential oil

3 drops sweet orange
essential oil

1. Put the essential oils in a small glass or ceramic bowl. Swirl the bowl around to blend the oils.

2. Put the cotton wick from the aromatherapy inhaler in the bowl and allow the wick to absorb the blend.

3. With a pair of tweezers, place the saturated wick into the aromatherapy inhaler and assemble. Snap or screw the cap into place. Affix a label to the inhaler.

4. Open the cap and inhale deeply through your nose as often as needed to stop feeling so overwhelmed.

SELF-CARE BOOST: Do you often say yes to things you really do not want to do or do not have time for? Saying yes all the time can lead to feeling overwhelmed. As a "yes person" myself, I have learned to default to the response, "Let me think about that and get back to you." That gives me time to figure out if I really have the interest and bandwidth to say yes. Try it out!

PANIC NO MORE ROLL-ON

This calming blend quiets the mind and promotes a sense of total relaxation. With lavender to ease jittery feelings, valerian to calm the overwhelming sense of tension and fear that typically accompanies panic, and Roman chamomile to gently release anxiety, this roll-on is ideal for application before a situation that might induce panic. Apply it if you start to feel frantic, too. The sooner you apply this blend, the faster you will feel those nervous, tense, fearful sensations evaporate. **TOPICAL, SAFE FOR AGES 6+, DO NOT USE IF PREGNANT, DO NOT USE WHILE DRIVING**

4 drops Roman chamomile essential oil
4 drops valerian essential oil
1 drop lavender essential oil
1¾ teaspoons jojoba oil

1. Using a fresh pipette for each oil, place the essential oils in a prelabeled 10-milliliter roller bottle. Add the jojoba oil.
2. Snap on the rollerball and screw on the cap. Shake until well-mixed.
3. Roll onto your wrists and other pulse points as needed to calm down.

SELF-CARE BOOST: One of the best ways to get grounded is to physically touch the ground! If the weather is right, go outside and take off your shoes. Proponents of "grounding" or "earthing" believe that putting our bare feet in contact with the ground allows our bodies to soak up the electromagnetic charge from the earth, which leads to overall balance and wellness.

FREEDOM FROM PANIC INHALER

This peaceful blend brings calming lavender and balancing ylang-ylang together with bergamot, which at once soothes, calms, and energizes you. This blend is ideal for situations when you must be alert and therefore need to avoid essential oils with stronger relaxation properties. If you are feeling tense or anxious but still need to power through your day, this is the blend for you. **DIRECT INHALATION, SAFE FOR AGES 2+, DO NOT USE IF PREGNANT**

9 drops lavender
essential oil

6 drops ylang-ylang
essential oil

6 drops bergamot
essential oil

1. Put the essential oils in a small glass or ceramic bowl. Swirl the bowl around to blend the oils.

2. Put the cotton wick from the aromatherapy inhaler in the bowl and allow the wick to absorb the blend.

3. With a pair of tweezers, place the saturated wick into the aromatherapy inhaler and assemble. Snap or screw the cap into place. Affix a label to the inhaler.

4. Open the cap and inhale deeply through your nose as often as needed to ease panic.

SELF-CARE BOOST: The negative thought loops that often accompany panic can take a serious psychological toll. It can be helpful to recognize that most negative thought loops are populated by hypothetical worst-case scenarios, which are unlikely to happen. So, when you catch yourself catastrophizing, ask yourself how probable each part of that imaginary chain of events really is. Then, try to replace the worst-case-scenario thoughts with best-case scenarios, which are more likely to happen anyway!

INSPIRE CONFIDENCE DIFFUSER BLEND

Bright, cheerful, and comforting, this delightful blend includes blue tansy and coriander, which are two of the best confidence-boosting essential oils. Sweet orange, spearmint, and lemon all lift your spirits and take your mind off unhelpful thoughts while simultaneously energizing you to take on the task at hand. **DIFFUSION, SAFE FOR AGES 2+**

24 drops sweet orange essential oil

16 drops lemon essential oil

12 drops coriander essential oil

12 drops spearmint essential oil

8 drops blue tansy essential oil

1. Put the essential oils in a small, dark-colored bottle. (If you are using a pipette to measure out the oils, use a new one for each essential oil—do not reuse.)

2. Cap the bottle tightly and swirl to blend the oils.

3. Add 8 to 10 drops of the blend to your diffuser, following the manufacturer's instructions. Label and store the remaining blend.

4. While the diffuser is running, simply relax and breathe while visualizing the best possible outcome.

DIRECT INHALATION OPTION: If you would like to attain greater confidence on the go, saturate the wick of an aromatherapy inhaler with 12 drops of this blend. (See Antianxiety Inhaler on page 79 for instructions.) Breathe deeply from your inhaler as often as needed.

SELF-CARE BOOST: The same anxiety that is hindering your sense of confidence often leads to shallow breathing, which makes you feel worse physically and mentally. Breathe deeply and intentionally while working to reframe your thoughts. If you are a visual person, try this meditation: Notice a self-doubt thought or word and, on each exhalation, imagine tying that word to a balloon and watching it float away into the sky.

UPLIFT AND UNWIND DIFFUSER BLEND

This peaceful blend helps you untangle mental knots while you continue activities or enjoy much-needed relaxation. With energetic sweet orange, soothing rose, and a wonderfully balancing base of sandalwood, it is ideal for grounding yourself when you are feeling agitated, anxious, or absolutely frantic. **DIFFUSION, SAFE FOR AGES 2+**

20 drops sandalwood essential oil

12 drops rose essential oil

8 drops sweet orange essential oil

1. Put the essential oils in a small, dark-colored bottle. (If you are using a pipette to measure out the oils, use a new one for each essential oil—do not reuse.)

2. Cap the bottle tightly and swirl to blend the oils.

3. Add 8 to 10 drops of the blend to your diffuser, following the manufacturer's instructions. Label and store the remaining blend.

4. While the diffuser is running, enjoy the aroma and recognize that you will make it through this day.

SELF-CARE BOOST: Engage in gentle exercise as often as you can, even if it happens in short bursts. A simple walk around the block can help you release some of the stress you are carrying in your body and mind.

BALANCE ROLL-ON

With soothing clary sage and relaxing notes of lavender and Roman chamomile, this balancing blend incorporates invigorating hints of grapefruit and sweet orange. When your mind is overloaded with rambling thoughts and your emotions are on edge, it can help you decompress quickly while putting things in perspective. **TOPICAL, SAFE FOR AGES 6+, DO NOT USE IF PREGNANT**

4 drops grapefruit essential oil

2 drops sweet orange essential oil

1 drop clary sage essential oil

1 drop lavender essential oil

1 drop Roman chamomile essential oil

1¾ teaspoons jojoba oil

1. Using a fresh pipette for each oil, place the essential oils in a prelabeled 10-milliliter roller bottle. Add the jojoba oil.

2. Snap on the rollerball and screw on the cap. Shake until well-mixed.

3. Roll onto your wrists and other pulse points as needed for a change in perspective.

SELF-CARE BOOST: Because stress can be an everyday issue, it is important to find a few healthy ways to handle the pressure. Listening to your favorite music, pausing to appreciate the sunset or the scent of rain, and treating your body to healthy food and drinks are a few simple methods for incorporating self-care into various aspects of your life.

DECOMPRESS DIFFUSER BLEND

Calming neroli, cypress, and spikenard mingle with balancing patchouli and a hint of inspiring orange in this beautifully fragrant blend. Individually, each of these oils is excellent for soothing frayed nerves; together, they can work wonders for your mental state. There is more to love: Studies have shown that neroli can help lower blood pressure and reduce cortisol levels associated with stress. **DIFFUSION, SAFE FOR AGES 2+, DO NOT USE IF PREGNANT OR BREASTFEEDING**

24 drops neroli essential oil

18 drops cypress essential oil

18 drops orange essential oil

16 drops patchouli essential oil

3 drops spikenard essential oil

1. Put the essential oils in a small, dark-colored bottle. (If you are using a pipette to measure out the oils, use a new one for each essential oil—do not reuse.)

2. Cap the bottle tightly and swirl to blend the oils.

3. Add 8 to 10 drops of the blend to your diffuser, following the manufacturer's instructions. Label and store the remaining blend.

4. While the diffuser is running, breathe deeply and relax away the tension.

SELF-CARE BOOST: Expose yourself to nature whenever you can. Studies show that spending time in natural settings can help our brains deal with stress and even provide a cognitive boost. Just 10 minutes spent breathing fresh air and appreciating nature's beauty can be beneficial.

MELT AWAY STRESS BODY OIL

This simple blend pairs the grounding scent of frankincense with the relaxing aroma of lavender. A wonderful synergy that helps your overworked mind and body, this oil is absorbed by both your olfactory system and your skin. This makes it great for daily moisturizing, massages, and adding to warm baths. **TOPICAL, SAFE FOR AGES 6+, DO NOT USE IF PREGNANT**

---

12 drops frankincense essential oil

6 drops lavender essential oil

4 ounces carrier oil

1. Put the essential oils in a 4-ounce, dark-colored bottle. Swirl to blend.

2. Add the carrier oil and cap the bottle tightly. Shake gently to mix.

3. For a relaxing bath, add 1 tablespoon of the oil to warm bathwater. To use as a moisturizer, rub about 1 teaspoon on your skin, using more or less as needed.

SELF-CARE BOOST: Unplug for a while each day. Spending every bit of your free time on your electronic device can make you even more stressed. If you need a nudge, download an app timer for your smartphone that alerts you when you have reached the limits you have set for yourself.

CLEAR VISION DIFFUSER BLEND

Confusion, anxiety, and overwhelm are some feelings associated with being stuck, wondering what to do next, and struggling to move forward when mental quicksand bogs you down. With bergamot to inspire you and melissa to dispel fatigue, irritability, and anxiety, plus peppermint for a hint of refreshing invigoration, this wonderful blend encourages the mind to find solutions where none existed before. **DIFFUSION, SAFE FOR AGES 2+, DO NOT USE IF PREGNANT OR BREASTFEEDING**

15 drops bergamot
    essential oil
15 drops melissa
    essential oil
15 drops peppermint
    essential oil

1. Put the essential oils in a small, dark-colored bottle. (If you are using a pipette to measure out the oils, use a new one for each essential oil—do not reuse.)

2. Cap the bottle tightly and swirl to blend the oils.

3. Add 8 to 10 drops of the blend to your diffuser, following the manufacturer's instructions. Label and store the remaining blend.

4. While the diffuser is running, enjoy the aroma and think about a goal or dream coming to fruition.

SELF-CARE BOOST: Feeling stuck can be a sign that you are heading toward exhaustion or burnout—or what I call "running on empty." If you frequently put others' needs ahead of your own, it is time to fill your own gas tank. While it might feel selfish, prioritizing your own needs puts you in a better position to help others later.

RELAX NOW ROLL-ON

Deeply soothing, this beautiful blend relies on lavender for its ability to calm frayed nerves, sweet orange to add a cheerful note, and patchouli to defuse irritated, angry feelings. Ylang-ylang contributes antidepressant properties while offering relief from the stress and anxiety that accompany tension. If you are feeling nervous, tense, or just plain stressed, reach for this peaceful, relaxing aromatherapy roll-on. **TOPICAL, SAFE FOR AGES 6+, DO NOT USE IF PREGNANT**

---

3 drops sweet orange essential oil

2 drops patchouli essential oil

1 drop lavender essential oil

1 drop ylang-ylang essential oil

1¾ teaspoons jojoba oil

1. Using a fresh pipette for each oil, put the essential oils in a prelabeled 10-milliliter roller bottle. Add the jojoba oil.

2. Snap on the rollerball and screw on the cap. Shake until well-mixed.

3. Roll onto your wrists and other pulse points as needed to relieve tension.

SELF-CARE BOOST: Tension and overwhelm often go hand in hand. If you can, take a break from whatever you are doing to renew your mind. A few tension-relieving stretches or a short walk while breathing deeply and deliberately can help defuse stress.

TENSION TAMER DIFFUSER BLEND

This blend brings several relaxing essential oils together and eases tension by encouraging your body and mind to relax. Spikenard, clary sage, and Roman chamomile are deeply calming, easing feelings of anger, aggression, stress, and restlessness. Melissa also shares these calming properties but offers a fresh, lemony scent that lightens the blend's fragrance. This deeply relaxing blend is ideal for diffusing at bedtime or while you are enjoying a warm bath. **DIFFUSION, SAFE FOR AGES 2+, DO NOT USE IF PREGNANT, DO NOT USE WHILE DRIVING**

20 drops clary sage
  essential oil
16 drops spikenard
  essential oil
12 drops melissa
  essential oil
12 drops Roman
  chamomile essential oil

1. Put the essential oils in a small, dark-colored bottle. (If you are using a pipette to measure out the oils, use a new one for each essential oil—do not reuse.)

2. Cap the bottle tightly and swirl to blend the oils.

3. Add 8 to 10 drops of the blend to your diffuser, following the manufacturer's instructions. Label and store the remaining blend.

4. While the diffuser is running, get ready for bed or relax in the tub.

SELF-CARE BOOST: It's a classic chicken-egg scenario: Which came first, the emotional tension or the physical tension? Whatever the cause, here is a quick meditation to help you release tension: Take a deep breath while focusing on the top of your head. When you exhale, release all the tension you are holding up there. On your next exhalation, move your attention down to your forehead, then your face, your jaw, your neck, and so on, until you have made your way down your entire body. You will probably feel muscles relax that you didn't even realize were tense!

CONTENTMENT ROLL-ON

Both copaiba and helichrysum essential oils are deeply healing when applied topically, making this roll-on a good one for wound healing, but that is just the beginning. Copaiba is especially beneficial for anxiety, depression, and underlying trauma, due to its high levels of β-caryophyllene. This blend lightens even the darkest moods, helping you deal with the stress and anxiety caused by fresh emotional trauma or deeply ingrained post-traumatic stress disorder (PTSD). Copaiba can lower your blood pressure if it is elevated, and helichrysum will help your mind relax. **TOPICAL, SAFE FOR AGES 6+**

6 drops copaiba
   essential oil
6 drops helichrysum
   essential oil
1¾ teaspoons jojoba oil

1. Using a fresh pipette for each oil, put the essential oils in a prelabeled 10-milliliter roller bottle. Add the jojoba oil.

2. Snap on the rollerball and screw on the cap. Shake until well-mixed.

3. Roll onto your wrists and other pulse points as needed.

4. As you apply the roll-on, breathe deeply and practice a grounding technique, such as touching an item with a soothing texture or listening to music that makes you feel good.

SELF-CARE BOOST: Many tools are available for survivors of trauma. Look into therapies like EMDR (eye movement desensitization and reprocessing) that help your brain reprocess traumatic memories and help you move forward.

POSITIVE RELIEF INHALER

Sweet, fresh lemon curbs negativity and promotes a positive outlook, and soothing lavender alleviates anxiety and helps relieve the nervousness and panic that often accompany deep-seated emotional trauma. Bergamot combats depression and anxiety while uplifting your mood and helping your mind find a calm, centered sense of focus. **DIRECT INHALATION, SAFE FOR AGES 6+, DO NOT USE IF PREGNANT**

4 drops bergamot
essential oil

4 drops lavender
essential oil

4 drops lemon essential oil

1. Put the essential oils in a small glass or ceramic bowl. Swirl the bowl around to blend the oils.

2. Put the cotton wick from the aromatherapy inhaler in the bowl and allow the wick to absorb the blend.

3. With a pair of tweezers, place the saturated wick into the aromatherapy inhaler and assemble. Snap or screw the cap into place. Affix a label to the inhaler.

4. Open the cap and inhale deeply through your nose as often as needed to improve your mood.

SELF-CARE BOOST: Deep emotional trauma and PTSD call for treatment from a knowledgeable mental health professional. It is so important to seek help if you are experiencing symptoms of trauma—especially if they are decreasing your quality of life. A therapist can help you process your emotions, deal with your symptoms, and increase your sense of well-being.

COMFORT ZONE DIFFUSER BLEND

Withdrawal comes with feelings of anxiety, tension, fear, negativity, and detachment. This blend addresses all of these unpleasant sensations while helping you deal with the physical sense of lethargy that often accompanies the emotional side of withdrawal. Do not worry if you are missing 1 or 2 of these oils; diffusing even 1 or 2 at a time can help move you toward a more positive mental space. **DIFFUSION, SAFE FOR AGES 2+, DO NOT USE IF PREGNANT**

24 drops grapefruit essential oil
12 drops lime essential oil
12 drops mandarin essential oil
9 drops lavender essential oil
6 drops holy basil essential oil

1. Put the essential oils in a small, dark-colored bottle. (If you are using a pipette to measure out the oils, use a new one for each essential oil—do not reuse.)

2. Cap the bottle tightly and swirl to blend the oils.

3. Add 8 to 10 drops of the blend to your diffuser, following the manufacturer's instructions. Label and store the remaining blend.

4. While the diffuser is running, sit back and allow yourself to experience the pleasant aroma.

DIRECT INHALATION OPTION: If you would like this blend to support you when you are out in the world, use 10 to 12 drops of this blend in an aromatherapy inhaler. (See Anti-anxiety Inhaler on page 79 for instructions.) Breathe deeply from your inhaler as often as needed.

SELF-CARE BOOST: We all need some alone time occasionally and a little social hibernation is often necessary, but feeling withdrawn and hopeless can be a sign of depression. If you notice that your symptoms are edging in that direction, reach out to a mental health professional. Getting ahead of these emotions can be extremely beneficial to helping you enjoy life again.

RELEASE WORRY ROLL-ON

With blue tansy to promote a sense of calm while easing your worried mind, this wonderfully complex blend incorporates lavender for its deeply soothing properties and sweet orange for its cheerful presence. When your brain is running in endless loops, reaching for this roll-on stops your "what if" thinking and helps you focus on positive solutions.

TOPICAL, SAFE FOR AGES 6+, DO NOT USE IF PREGNANT, DO NOT USE WITH DRUGS METABOLIZED BY CYP2D6

6 drops lavender essential oil

4 drops sweet orange essential oil

2 drops blue tansy essential oil

1¾ teaspoons jojoba oil

1. Using a fresh pipette for each oil, place the essential oils in a prelabeled 10-milliliter roller bottle. Add the jojoba oil.

2. Snap on the rollerball and screw on the cap. Shake until well-mixed.

3. Roll onto wrists and other pulse points as needed while breathing deeply and thinking about whether there are any productive steps you can take right now.

SELF-CARE BOOST: Worries are often unfounded fears, but that does not mean you should ignore them. When we let worries float around in our head, they can grow to a massive size. Writing down your worries can take the power out of them, so try making a list of the thoughts jumping around in your head and include any actionable solutions. When you see them in the light of day, you might find that your fears are not so scary after all!

PEACE-IN-A-BOTTLE DIFFUSER BLEND

This peaceful blend is deeply grounding and wonderfully restful, leaving your body feeling more relaxed and encouraging your mind to stop the unproductive chatter that accompanies worry. Sandalwood, cedarwood, and lavender help release anxiety and stress, too, making this blend ideal for times when you are ill at ease. **DIFFUSION, SAFE FOR AGES 2+, DO NOT USE IF PREGNANT**

30 drops sandalwood
   essential oil
15 drops lavender
   essential oil
3 drops cedarwood
   essential oil

1. Put the essential oils in a small, dark-colored bottle. (If you are using a pipette to measure out the oils, use a new one for each essential oil—do not reuse.)

2. Cap the bottle tightly and swirl to blend the oils.

3. Add 8 to 10 drops of the blend to your diffuser, following the manufacturer's instructions. Label and store the remaining blend.

4. While the diffuser is running, breathe in feelings of peace and breathe out stress.

BATH OPTION: This blend makes a wonderful massage or bath oil. If you would like to try it, combine the essential oils in a 4-ounce bottle and fill with about 4 ounces of your favorite carrier oil. Cap the bottle and shake gently to blend. Use 1 tablespoon in a warm bath or 1 teaspoon for a soothing massage.

SELF-CARE BOOST: One fascinating study found that setting aside a specific time for worry can help reduce the overall time spent worrying. Try setting aside 15 to 30 minutes specifically for thinking about things that bother you and deciding on productive ways to cope. Tell yourself to postpone worrying until your scheduled time, and if you catch yourself in a downward spiral, remind yourself that you will revisit those thoughts when it is time to do so.

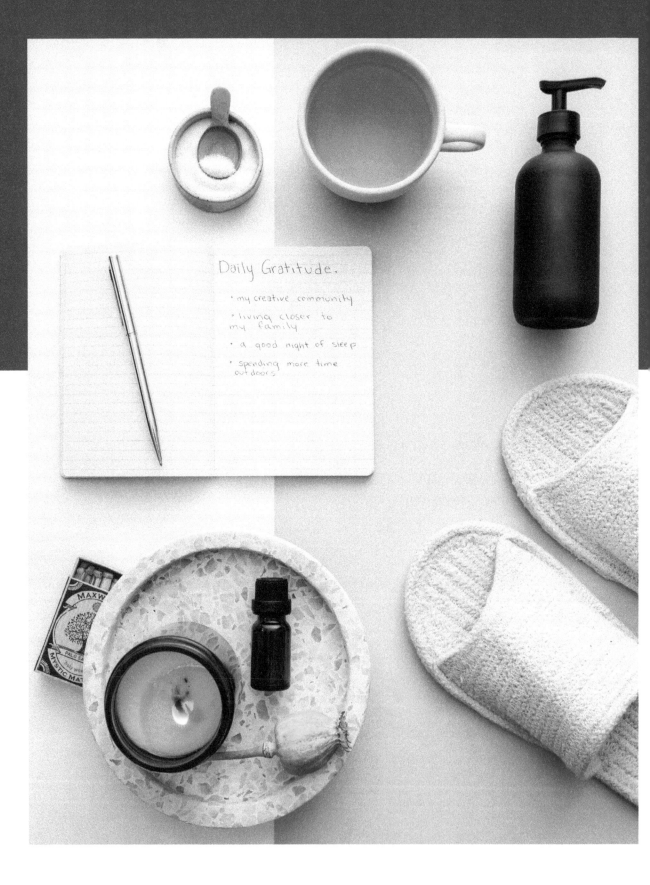

Daily Gratitude.

• my creative community
• living closer to my family
• a good night of sleep
• spending more time outdoors

06

Mental Well-Being

We humans are intricate beings, with minds that require a balance of stimulation and relaxation. Aromatherapy can bolster your efforts to enjoy productive work and satisfying creative pursuits, and it can support your efforts to relax and unwind when the time comes. Most of the blends in this chapter are designed for direct inhalation or use in a diffuser, so they are easier to fit into your life. You will notice plenty of stimulating herb and citrus oils in blends for creativity, memory, and more, and relaxing options like vetiver, valerian, and lavender in remedies designed to help you enjoy fulfilling downtime.

CREATIVE BOOST INHALER

When it is time to engage in creative work, this blend can help. With lemon and frankincense to enhance focus, spearmint to erase mental fog, and rosemary to boost overall mental performance, this inhaler is easy to reach for anytime you would like to bolster creativity.

DIRECT INHALATION, SAFE FOR AGES 10+

3 drops frankincense essential oil

3 drops lemon essential oil

2 drops rosemary essential oil

2 drops spearmint essential oil

1. Put the essential oils in a small glass or ceramic bowl. Swirl the bowl around to blend the oils.

2. Put the cotton wick from the aromatherapy inhaler in the bowl and allow the wick to absorb the blend.

3. With a pair of tweezers, place the saturated wick into the aromatherapy inhaler and assemble. Snap or screw the cap into place. Affix a label to the inhaler.

4. Open the cap and inhale deeply through your nose to enhance creativity as often as needed.

SELF-CARE BOOST: Have you ever noticed that some of your best ideas come to you while you are showering? When you give your mind space to relax, your creativity gets a boost. Try inhaling this blend before stepping into a warm shower and see what happens.

INSPIRING ATMOSPHERE ROOM SPRAY

With energizing notes of pine and bergamot plus a refreshing touch of peppermint, this delightful room spray also contains eucalyptus to enhance focus. Together, these essential oils help clear mental fog, enhance your sense of alertness, and promote openness to creative intuition. If inspiration seems difficult to find, refreshing your space with this spray can help. **ATMOSPHERIC DIFFUSION, SAFE FOR AGES 2+, DO NOT USE IF PREGNANT OR BREASTFEEDING**

12 drops eucalyptus essential oil

12 drops bergamot essential oil

8 drops pine essential oil

4 drops peppermint essential oil

1 teaspoon Himalayan salt or sea salt

3¾ ounces distilled water

1. Put the essential oils in a bottle that can be fitted with a spray top. (If you are using a pipette to measure out the oils, use a new one for each essential oil—do not reuse.) Swirl for a few seconds to blend.

2. Using a funnel, pour the salt into the bottle and swirl again to blend the essential oils with the salt.

3. Again, using a funnel, pour the distilled water into the bottle.

4. Affix the spray top, tighten it securely, and shake to blend well. Label the bottle.

5. It is okay to use this blend immediately, but if you would like to enjoy a stronger fragrance, let the bottle rest for 2 days before use.

6. Spritz into the air to promote an atmosphere of inspiration.

SELF-CARE BOOST: Exercise is a great way to increase circulation to the brain, so be sure to enjoy regular walks, runs, or workouts. Your entire body and mind will thank you.

INSPIRE INNER VISION DIFFUSER BLEND

If you find yourself struggling with creative blocks or self-doubt, this blend can make a difference. With sandalwood to instill a sense of confident self-awareness, frankincense to bolster concentration, and ylang-ylang to inspire you while fostering a stress-free atmosphere, this diffusion is one to enjoy anytime you would like to get into a state of flow.

DIFFUSION, SAFE FOR AGES 2+

10 drops frankincense essential oil

10 drops sandalwood essential oil

10 drops ylang-ylang essential oil

1. Put the essential oils in a small, dark-colored bottle. (If you are using a pipette to measure out the oils, use a new one for each essential oil—do not reuse.)

2. Cap the bottle tightly and swirl to blend the oils.

3. Add 8 to 10 drops of the blend to your diffuser, following the manufacturer's instructions. Label and store the remaining blend.

4. While the diffuser is running, engage in activities calling on you to be creative.

DIRECT INHALATION OPTION: If you would like to use this remedy on the go, use 8 to 10 drops of this blend in an aromatherapy inhaler. (See Antianxiety Inhaler on page 79 for instructions.) Breathe deeply from your inhaler as often as needed.

SELF-CARE BOOST: Wracking your brain tends to be counterproductive, so give yourself permission to stop thinking. While you are relaxing, your brain can find solutions to problems all on its own. Run your diffuser with a creativity-stimulating blend, sit back, and let the magic happen.

ENTHUSIASM DIFFUSER BLEND

This stimulating blend enhances your ability to concentrate and focus while cultivating a joyful, energetic atmosphere. If you are missing mandarin in your essential oil stash, feel free to substitute with any other citrus oil. The scent will stimulate your senses and the overall effect will be similar. **DIFFUSION, SAFE FOR AGES 2+, DO NOT USE IF BREASTFEEDING, DO NOT USE WITH DRUGS METABOLIZED BY CYP2B6**

12 drops frankincense essential oil
12 drops mandarin essential oil
6 drops lemongrass essential oil

1. Put the essential oils in a small, dark-colored bottle. (If you are using a pipette to measure out the oils, use a new one for each essential oil—do not reuse.)

2. Cap the bottle tightly and swirl to blend the oils.

3. Add 8 to 10 drops of the blend to your diffuser, following the manufacturer's instructions. Label and store the remaining blend.

4. While the diffuser is running, put your renewed concentration and focus to work.

DIRECT INHALATION OPTION: If you would like to use this remedy on the go, use 8 to 10 drops of this blend in an aromatherapy inhaler. (See Antianxiety Inhaler on page 79 for instructions.) Breathe deeply from your inhaler as often as needed.

SELF-CARE BOOST: Move a little more! Studies suggest that a quick walk—as little as 10 minutes—can help perk you up better than a sugary snack. Try pairing this diffusion with some easy at-home exercises, like jumping jacks or mountain climbers. Dancing in your kitchen counts, too!

QUICK PICK-ME-UP INHALER

Lime is used to promote better energy flow throughout the body; its cheerful, refreshing aroma is wonderfully restorative. Grapefruit bolsters energy, whereas peppermint helps beat fatigue. Together, this invigorating trio helps boost your spirits while encouraging you to get up, get moving, and take care of your to-do list. **DIRECT INHALATION, SAFE FOR AGES 6+, DO NOT USE IF PREGNANT OR BREASTFEEDING**

6 drops grapefruit essential oil

3 drops peppermint essential oil

3 drops lime essential oil

1. Put the essential oils in a small glass or ceramic bowl. Swirl the bowl around to blend the oils.

2. Put the cotton wick from the aromatherapy inhaler in the bowl and allow the wick to absorb the blend.

3. With a pair of tweezers, place the saturated wick into the aromatherapy inhaler and assemble. Snap or screw the cap into place. Affix a label to the inhaler.

4. Open the cap and inhale deeply through your nose to enjoy a quick energy boost whenever you need it.

SELF-CARE BOOST: Crashing after meals or snacks? If so, check your sugar intake. While sugar might give you a quick jolt of energy, it is usually followed by a crash. Avoiding products with added sugar (which is often disguised by other names) is a good first step in preventing this. It takes an effort to ditch the sweet stuff, but when you do, you will notice that your energy levels remain more stable throughout the day.

ENERGIZING ROOM SPRAY

This revitalizing blend pairs the joyful scent of lemon with stimulating rosemary and basil. Uplifting and refreshing, this trio of oils work to enhance mental focus while providing an encouraging sense of energy in your space. Like other blends that contain rosemary, this one promotes alertness so well that you might want to avoid using it within a few hours of bedtime. **ATMOSPHERIC DIFFUSION, SAFE FOR AGES 2+, DO NOT USE IF PREGNANT OR BREASTFEEDING**

18 drops rosemary
essential oil
12 drops lemon
essential oil
6 drops basil essential oil
1 teaspoon Himalayan salt
or sea salt
3¾ ounces
distilled water

1. Put the essential oils in a bottle that can be fitted with a spray top. (If you are using a pipette to measure out the oils, use a new one for each essential oil—do not reuse.) Swirl for a few seconds to blend.

2. Using a funnel, pour the salt into the bottle and swirl again to blend the essential oils with the salt.

3. Again, using a funnel, pour the distilled water into the bottle.

4. Affix the spray top, tighten it securely, and shake the blend well. Label the bottle.

5. It is okay to use this blend immediately, but if you would like to enjoy a stronger fragrance, let the bottle rest for 2 days before use.

6. Spritz into the air to promote an uplifting, energetic atmosphere.

SELF-CARE BOOST: How is your hydration level? If you are not drinking enough water, you are likely to feel lethargic. Drink water throughout the day and you will probably find that your mood, energy, and brain function improve.

TIME-OUT ROLL-ON

Both soothing and uplifting, this blend includes lavender to encourage your mind and body to relax a bit, plus sage and rosemary to keep you mentally alert so that you can continue your day. Wonderfully grounding yet ideal for fighting fatigue, this refreshing roll-on is a quick antidote to exhaustion when you do not have time to fully unwind. **TOPICAL, SAFE FOR AGES 2+, DO NOT USE IF PREGNANT OR BREASTFEEDING**

5 drops lavender
essential oil

2 drops sage
essential oil

2 drops rosemary
essential oil

1¾ teaspoons
jojoba oil

1. Using a fresh pipette for each oil, place the essential oils in a prelabeled 10-milliliter roller bottle. Add the jojoba oil.

2. Snap on the rollerball and screw on the cap. Shake until well-mixed.

3. Roll onto your wrists and other pulse points as needed.

SELF-CARE BOOST: Take a 15-minute time-out and treat yourself to a mini-retreat: Make yourself a warm cup of tea, grab a fluffy blanket, put your electronic devices out of reach, and dab on this roll-on. Do absolutely nothing other than sit and enjoy your blanket and your tea.

REVIVE DIFFUSER BLEND

With clary sage to ground you, this complex blend also includes lemon, pine, and rosemary to energize your mind. Thyme adds an encouraging note whereas pine provides uplifting presence. When you are feeling mentally burdened and physically spent, this blend can provide an energizing boost while improving your outlook. **DIFFUSION, SAFE FOR AGES 2+, DO NOT USE IF PREGNANT, DO NOT USE WITH BLOOD THINNERS**

12 drops rosemary essential oil

9 drops bergamot essential oil

9 drops pine essential oil

9 drops thyme essential oil

6 drops clary sage essential oil

3 drops lemon essential oil

1. Put the essential oils in a small, dark-colored bottle. (If you are using a pipette to measure out the oils, use a new one for each essential oil—do not reuse.)

2. Cap the bottle tightly and swirl to blend the oils.

3. Add 8 to 10 drops of the blend to your diffuser, following the manufacturer's instructions. Label and store the remaining blend.

4. While the diffuser is running, tackle that thing that requires your mental energy.

DIRECT INHALATION OPTION: If you would like to use this remedy on the go, use 8 to 10 drops of this blend in an aromatherapy inhaler. (See Antianxiety Inhaler on page 79 for instructions.) Breathe deeply from your inhaler to revive yourself as often as needed.

SELF-CARE BOOST: When you are exhausted but do not have time to rest, turn on some uplifting music. Even if you are not really paying attention to it, it will give you a mental boost and make your work feel more bearable.

LIFT ME UP ROLL-ON

Clarifying, harmonizing, and balancing, this refreshing blend helps restore your energy with spirited notes of mandarin and grapefruit. Bergamot mint supports mental clarity, whereas rose geranium encourages a sense of overall well-being. This blend is wonderful anytime, but it really shines when negative situations contribute to feelings of exhaustion. **TOPICAL, SAFE FOR AGES 6+**

5 drops bergamot mint
   essential oil
2 drops rose geranium
   essential oil
1 drop mandarin
   essential oil
1 drop grapefruit
   essential oil
1¾ teaspoons
   jojoba oil

1. Using a fresh pipette for each oil, put the essential oils in a prelabeled 10-milliliter roller bottle. Add the jojoba oil.

2. Snap on the rollerball and screw on the cap. Shake until well-mixed.

3. Roll onto your wrists and other pulse points as needed.

SELF-CARE BOOST: If you are frequently exhausted and you cannot quite figure out why, consider visiting your health-care practitioner to rule out an underlying cause. Frequent exhaustion can be a sign of thyroid dysfunction or anemia, so it is a good idea to get checked out.

LIVELY MIND DIFFUSER BLEND

Hyssop contributes warm, woody notes to this uplifting, energizing blend while supporting mental clarity and easing fatigue. Grapefruit and mandarin further energize the mind, inspiring happiness and resetting your inner sense of balance. This blend is helpful anytime that mental fatigue leaves you feeling discouraged, bored, or simply out of whack. **DIFFUSION, SAFE FOR AGES 2+, DO NOT USE IF PREGNANT OR BREASTFEEDING**

20 drops hyssop
essential oil
10 drops grapefruit
essential oil
10 drops mandarin
essential oil

1. Put the essential oils in a small, dark-colored bottle. (If you are using a pipette to measure out the oils, use a new one for each essential oil—do not reuse.)

2. Cap the bottle tightly and swirl to blend the oils.

3. Add 8 to 10 drops of the blend to your diffuser, following the manufacturer's instructions. Label and store the remaining blend.

4. While the diffuser is running, allow your mental fatigue to melt away.

DIRECT INHALATION OPTION: If you would like to use this remedy on the go, use 8 to 10 drops of this blend in an aromatherapy inhaler. (See Antianxiety Inhaler on page 79 for instructions.) Breathe deeply from your inhaler as often as needed to renew your mental clarity.

SELF-CARE BOOST: Check your daily and weekly schedules. Are you overcommitting? If so, the continuous cognitive strain could be contributing to your mental fatigue. To avoid burnout, cut back on your commitments.

PRODUCTIVITY DIFFUSER BLEND

With bold notes of peppermint and rosemary tempered by refreshing balsam fir and uplifting bergamot, this exhilarating diffusion clears your mind and helps you continue with essential tasks when you have no time to stop and rest. Try it anytime you would like help with concentration or energy. **DIFFUSION, SAFE FOR AGES 2+, DO NOT USE IF PREGNANT OR BREASTFEEDING**

16 drops peppermint essential oil

16 drops rosemary essential oil

12 drops bergamot essential oil

4 drops balsam fir essential oil

1. Put the essential oils in a small, dark-colored bottle. (If you are using a pipette to measure out the oils, use a new one for each essential oil—do not reuse.)

2. Cap the bottle tightly and swirl to blend the oils.

3. Add 8 to 10 drops of the blend to your diffuser, following the manufacturer's instructions. Label and store the remaining blend.

4. While the diffuser is running, focus on whatever needs your attention.

DIRECT INHALATION OPTION: If you would like to use this remedy on the go, use 8 to 10 drops of this blend in an aromatherapy inhaler. (See Antianxiety Inhaler on page 79 for instructions.) Breathe deeply from your inhaler to boost your productivity as often as needed.

SELF-CARE BOOST: Being well-organized can help ease ongoing mental fatigue. Set aside time for tidying up, updating your calendar, and creating to-do lists. When you have everything in place, you will find that it is easier to stay motivated, focused, and productive.

EFFICIENCY INHALER

This energizing blend clears away mental cobwebs so it is easier to focus, study, work, or simply continue making your way through a day packed with not-so-fun errands and obligations. When you are feeling mentally overloaded and you would like to throw in the towel, this inhaler can be a lifesaver. **DIRECT INHALATION, SAFE FOR AGES 12+**

6 drops lemon
essential oil
4 drops rosemary
essential oil
2 drops basil
essential oil

1. Put the essential oils in a small glass or ceramic bowl. Swirl the bowl around to blend the oils.

2. Put the cotton wick from the aromatherapy inhaler in the bowl and allow the wick to absorb the blend.

3. With a pair of tweezers, place the saturated wick into the aromatherapy inhaler and assemble. Snap or screw the cap into place. Affix a label to the inhaler.

4. Open the cap and inhale deeply through your nose to enjoy a burst of mental energy as often as needed.

SELF-CARE BOOST: Just like you would not wait until your car's gas tank was completely empty before you refill it, you cannot put off prioritizing self-care until you are completely exhausted. Stay ahead of the game by taking quick daily strolls, prioritizing weekend relaxation, and taking vacations when you can.

DEEP FLOW DIFFUSER BLEND

With rosemary and sage to ground you and improve focus while promoting a sense of calm confidence, this marvelous blend offers an invigorating hint of lemon and just a touch of woody, relaxing cypress. This blend is ideal for those times when you would like to dig deeply and produce some of your very best work. **DIFFUSION, SAFE FOR AGES 2+, DO NOT USE IF PREGNANT OR BREASTFEEDING**

10 drops cypress essential oil

10 drops lemon essential oil

10 drops rosemary essential oil

10 drops sage essential oil

1. Put the essential oils in a small, dark-colored bottle. (If you are using a pipette to measure out the oils, use a new one for each essential oil—do not reuse.)

2. Cap the bottle tightly and swirl to blend the oils.

3. Add 8 to 10 drops of the blend to your diffuser, following the manufacturer's instructions. Label and store the remaining blend.

4. While the diffuser is running, create your masterpiece in whatever form it takes.

DIRECT INHALATION OPTION: If you would like to use this remedy on the go, use 8 to 10 drops of this blend in an aromatherapy inhaler. (See Antianxiety Inhaler on page 79 for instructions.) Breathe deeply from your inhaler as often as needed to get into the flow.

SELF-CARE BOOST: Distractions force you to spend more time on tasks, so eliminate them if you can by finding ways to work undisturbed. Put your phone away and turn off annoying message pop-ups on your computer. You will focus better and, in the end, you will have more time to spend on things you enjoy.

CONCENTRATION INHALER

Together, rosemary, basil, and cypress create a blend that promotes deep concentration while enhancing memory and sharpening your mind. This blend offers a balancing, calming effect while keeping you mentally energized. Use this inhaler anytime you would like to focus better. **DIRECT INHALATION, SAFE FOR AGES 10+, DO NOT USE IF PREGNANT OR BREASTFEEDING**

4 drops basil essential oil

4 drops cypress
  essential oil

4 drops rosemary
  essential oil

1. Put the essential oils in a small glass or ceramic bowl. Swirl the bowl around to blend the oils.

2. Put the cotton wick from the aromatherapy inhaler in the bowl and allow the wick to absorb the blend.

3. With a pair of tweezers, place the saturated wick into the aromatherapy inhaler and assemble. Snap or screw the cap into place. Affix a label to the inhaler.

4. Open the cap and inhale deeply through your nose to increase focus as often as needed.

SELF-CARE BOOST: If you have trouble focusing at work, spend 10 minutes at home each day to practice a mindfulness meditation. In time, your ability to focus and concentrate during your workday will improve.

GET IN THE ZONE ROOM SPRAY

This blend is perfect for refreshing your space prior to a meeting or study session. With rosemary to maximize mental acuity, grapefruit to increase attention span, and lime to promote a sense of positive energy, this spray doubles as a delightfully scented all-natural air freshener. **ATMOSPHERIC DIFFUSION, SAFE FOR AGES 2+**

12 drops grapefruit essential oil

12 drops lime essential oil

12 drops rosemary essential oil

1 teaspoon Himalayan salt or sea salt

3¾ ounces distilled water

1. Put the essential oils in a bottle that can be fitted with a spray top. (If you are using a pipette to measure out the oils, use a new one for each essential oil—do not reuse.) Swirl for a few seconds to blend.

2. Using a funnel, pour the salt into the bottle and swirl again to blend the essential oils with the salt.

3. Again, using a funnel, pour the distilled water into the bottle.

4. Affix the spray top, tighten it securely, and shake the blend well. Label the bottle.

5. It is okay to use this blend immediately, but if you would like to enjoy a stronger fragrance, let the bottle rest for 2 days before use.

6. Spritz into the air to promote an atmosphere of concentration.

CLARITY AND VISION DIFFUSER BLEND

Euphoric notes of lemon, spearmint, and frankincense mingle beautifully with grounding rosemary in this refreshing blend. Relaxing yet energizing, the oils in this blend are perfect for conceptual work or simply for allowing you to flex your creative muscle. **DIFFUSION, SAFE FOR AGES 2+, DO NOT USE IF PREGNANT OR BREASTFEEDING**

12 drops frankincense essential oil
8 drops lemon essential oil
8 drops spearmint essential oil
4 drops rosemary essential oil

1. Put the essential oils in a small, dark-colored bottle. (If you are using a pipette to measure out the oils, use a new one for each essential oil—do not reuse.)
2. Cap the bottle tightly and swirl to blend the oils.
3. Add 8 to 10 drops of the blend to your diffuser, following the manufacturer's instructions. Label and store the remaining blend.
4. While the diffuser is running, allow your imagination to come to the forefront.

DIRECT INHALATION OPTION: If you would like to use this remedy on the go, use 8 to 10 drops of this blend in an aromatherapy inhaler. (See Antianxiety Inhaler on page 79 for instructions.) Breathe deeply from your inhaler as often as needed to get your gears turning.

SELF-CARE BOOST: When you need to plan and brainstorm, try thinking in pictures instead of words. Visual thinking is an imaginative approach to problem-solving that you might enjoy. For example, try this exercise: Visualize your priorities with a simple sketch of a bar graph. Use rough estimates for the percentages of time you're spending on different things.

SPARK IMAGINATION INHALER

Maximize your imagination's abilities with this uplifting blend. With joyful notes of jasmine and sweet orange, the blend includes just the right amount of patchouli to encourage free, creative thinking. When you are feeling blocked by doubt, stress, or negativity in general, you will find that this inhaler can be an effective antidote. **DIRECT INHALATION, SAFE FOR AGES 2+, DO NOT USE WITH BLOOD THINNERS**

4 drops jasmine essential oil

4 drops patchouli essential oil

4 drops sweet orange essential oil

1. Put the essential oils in a small glass or ceramic bowl. Swirl the bowl around to blend the oils.

2. Place the cotton wick from the aromatherapy inhaler in the bowl and allow the wick to absorb the blend.

3. With a pair of tweezers, place the saturated wick into the aromatherapy inhaler and assemble. Snap or screw the cap into place. Affix a label to the inhaler.

4. Open the cap and inhale deeply through your nose to encourage imaginative thoughts as often as needed.

SELF-CARE BOOST: Feeling uninventive or uncreative? An overloaded schedule smothers imagination, so be sure to take time to relax, unwind, and do things you enjoy. It is far easier to prevent burnout than to recover from it.

BRAINSTORM SESH ROOM SPRAY

This balancing blend includes relaxing notes of lavender, geranium, and rose geranium, a trio that also helps reduce headaches. Sandalwood introduces a grounding, meditative touch and peppermint renews alertness. Whether you are brainstorming with a group or forming ideas alone, this refreshing, spirited room spray helps create the ideal atmosphere for enhanced mental performance and maximum creativity. **ATMOSPHERIC DIFFUSION, SAFE FOR AGES 2+, DO NOT USE IF PREGNANT OR BREASTFEEDING**

9 drops lavender essential oil

9 drops lemon essential oil

6 drops peppermint essential oil

6 drops sandalwood essential oil

3 drops geranium essential oil

3 drops rose geranium essential oil

1 teaspoon Himalayan salt or sea salt

3¾ ounces distilled water

1. Put the essential oils in a bottle that can be fitted with a spray top. (If you are using a pipette to measure out the oils, use a new one for each essential oil—do not reuse.) Swirl for a few seconds to blend.

2. Using a funnel, pour the salt into the bottle and swirl again to blend the essential oils with the salt.

3. Again, using a funnel, pour the distilled water into the bottle.

4. Affix the spray top, tighten it securely, and shake the blend well. Label the bottle.

5. It is okay to use this blend immediately, but if you prefer a stronger fragrance, let the bottle rest for 2 days before use.

6. Spritz into the air to promote an atmosphere of creativity.

SELF-CARE BOOST: Too much information creates mental clutter that gets in the way of your naturally creative thought process. Develop a regular habit of taking time away from media, phones, computers, TVs, and other sources of endless information. A daily habit of no screen time is most beneficial, but even an occasional "digital detox" will help refresh your imagination.

QUIET MIND BODY OIL

This versatile massage oil brings cheerful ylang-ylang together with reassuring vetiver and relaxing lavender, helping you release your worries, stop troublesome mental chatter, and ease physical tension. The delicious aroma promotes an instant sense of relaxation that encourages you to drift off peacefully. **TOPICAL, SAFE FOR AGES 2+, DO NOT USE IF PREGNANT**

8 drops ylang-ylang
essential oil

4 drops lavender
essential oil

4 drops vetiver essential oil

4 ounces carrier oil

1. Put the essential oils in a 4-ounce, dark-colored bottle. Swirl to blend.

2. Add the carrier oil and cap the bottle tightly. Shake gently to mix.

3. For a relaxing bath, add 1 tablespoon of the oil to warm bathwater. To use as a moisturizer, rub about 1 teaspoon on your skin, using more or less as needed.

ACUPRESSURE TIP: Settle your mind by using acupressure on your heart channel points, which you will find on the inner arm. Heart 7 (located in the wrist crease just inside the tendon that runs to your pinky finger) is a great point for settling the spirit. Dab a few drops of this blend on the point and apply moderate pressure for up to 90 seconds.

SELF-CARE BOOST: Try pairing this comforting blend with a cup of chamomile or lavender tea to help you get into a more restful state.

RESTFUL DIFFUSER BLEND

This deeply soothing blend eases the overthinking that tends to accompany insomnia while encouraging your nervous system to slow its pace in preparation for sleep. Whether you are anxiously working on a problem or thinking about the day's challenges, this restful blend can help. **DIFFUSION, SAFE FOR AGES 2+, DO NOT USE IF PREGNANT**

5 drops lavender
    essential oil
3 drops geranium
    essential oil
3 drops vetiver essential oil
2 drops cedarwood
    essential oil
2 drops frankincense
    essential oil

1. Put the essential oils in a small, dark-colored bottle. (If you are using a pipette to measure out the oils, use a new one for each essential oil—do not reuse.)
2. Cap the bottle tightly and swirl to blend the oils.
3. Add 8 to 10 drops of the blend to your diffuser, following the manufacturer's instructions. Label and store the remaining blend.
4. While the diffuser is running, sit back and relax.

DIRECT INHALATION OPTION: If you would like this remedy to be on call at your bedside, use 8 to 10 drops of this blend in an aromatherapy inhaler. (See Antianxiety Inhaler on page 79 for instructions.) Breathe deeply from your inhaler before settling in for sleep and as needed throughout the night.

SELF-CARE BOOST: Sleep experts recommend shutting off all electronic devices at least half an hour before bed, since the blue light from screens stimulates wakefulness. You may find it very helpful to reach for a paper book if you need entertainment in the late evenings.

DREAMTIME PILLOW SPRAY

Deeply calming clary sage, lavender, and valerian combine with balancing marjoram, creating a hypnotic fragrance with a soothing, sedating effect. This peaceful blend can help you get past troublesome thoughts that keep you awake. If stress, anxiety, and tension are part of the problem, this blend will help you relax physically and mentally. **ATMOSPHERIC DIFFUSION, SAFE FOR AGES 2+, DO NOT USE IF PREGNANT, DO NOT USE WHILE DRIVING**

10 drops clary sage essential oil

10 drops lavender essential oil

10 drops marjoram essential oil

5 drops valerian essential oil

3¾ ounces witch hazel

1. Put the essential oils in a bottle that can be fitted with a spray top. (If you are using a pipette to measure out the oils, use a new one for each essential oil—do not reuse.) Swirl for a few seconds to blend.

2. Using a funnel, pour the witch hazel into the bottle.

3. Affix the spray top, tighten it securely, and shake to blend well. Label the bottle.

4. Spritz your sheets and pillowcase with the spray a few minutes before bedtime.

DIFFUSION OPTION: You can use this same aromatherapy blend in your diffuser. Blend the essential oils together in a small, dark-colored bottle and add 8 to 10 drops to your diffuser before hitting the pillow.

SELF-CARE BOOST: Melatonin supplements reduce the amount of time it takes to fall asleep while promoting deeper, more restful slumber without leaving you groggy the next day. Talk with your health-care practitioner about this natural supplement to see if it might be right for you.

BALANCE DIFFUSER BLEND

Tranquil vetiver adds just the right amount of earthiness to this wonderful diffusion, which incorporates soothing florals, revitalizing citrus, and a warm note of cedarwood. Together, these oils promote a sense of relaxed mental awareness that encourages you to cultivate mindfulness. **DIFFUSION, SAFE FOR AGES 2+**

20 drops sweet orange essential oil

16 drops rose or rose geranium essential oil

10 drops cedarwood essential oil

4 drops vetiver essential oil

1. Put the essential oils in a small, dark-colored bottle. (If you are using a pipette to measure out the oils, use a new one for each essential oil—do not reuse.)

2. Cap the bottle tightly and swirl to blend the oils.

3. Add 8 to 10 drops of the blend to your diffuser, following the manufacturer's instructions. Label and store the remaining blend.

4. While the diffuser is running, settle down for meditation or contemplation.

DIRECT INHALATION OPTION: If you would like to use this remedy on the go, use 8 to 10 drops of this blend in an aromatherapy inhaler. (See Antianxiety Inhaler on page 79 for instructions.) Breathe deeply from your inhaler as often as needed to cultivate mindfulness in your daily activities.

SELF-CARE BOOST: If you are new to meditation and you have trouble focusing, consider clearing your mind before meditating. This is easier than it sounds: Just take a few minutes to write down whatever is on your mind. When those thoughts interrupt you while you are meditating, remind yourself that you can look at your list after your session.

SPIRITUAL RETREAT DIFFUSER BLEND

With grounding notes of frankincense and myrrh plus a lighter, more refreshing note of cedarwood, this soothing blend is ideal for creating a peaceful, spiritual atmosphere for meditation. These wonderfully harmonizing essential oils ease tension and help you unwind, making this diffusion ideal for relaxation as well as mindfulness. **DIFFUSION, SAFE FOR AGES 2+, DO NOT USE IF PREGNANT OR BREASTFEEDING**

12 drops cedarwood
essential oil
12 drops frankincense
essential oil
12 drops myrrh
essential oil

1. Put the essential oils in a small, dark-colored bottle. (If you are using a pipette to measure out the oils, use a new one for each essential oil—do not reuse.)

2. Cap the bottle tightly and swirl to blend the oils.

3. Add 8 to 10 drops of the blend to your diffuser, following the manufacturer's instructions. Label and store the remaining blend.

4. While the diffuser is running, simply enjoy the moments of tranquility.

DIRECT INHALATION OPTION: If you would like to use this remedy on the go, use 8 to 10 drops of this blend in an aromatherapy inhaler. (See Antianxiety Inhaler on page 79 for instructions.) Breathe deeply from your inhaler to add a touch of tranquility to your day.

ACUPRESSURE TIP: Kidney 1, which is located on the bottom of the foot, is the most grounding acupressure point on the body. To enhance your meditation practice, first do a gentle acupressure massage on this point for up to 90 seconds. This will bring your energy down and get you out of your head.

SELF-CARE BOOST: Before you sit down to meditate, minimize the potential for distraction by silencing your phone and other electronic devices.

RELAXED CLARITY DIFFUSER BLEND

This uplifting blend relaxes your mind while reducing outside distractions so you can focus on mindfulness. With cedarwood to enhance mental clarity, sandalwood to balance emotions, and lemon to promote fresh perspective, this blend is a wonderful one to use for meditation or anytime you would like to create a calm atmosphere in your home. **DIFFUSION, SAFE FOR AGES 2+**

20 drops sandalwood essential oil
10 drops cedarwood essential oil
10 drops lemon essential oil

1. Put the essential oils in a small, dark-colored bottle. (If you are using a pipette to measure out the oils, use a new one for each essential oil—do not reuse.)
2. Cap the bottle tightly and swirl to blend the oils.
3. Add 8 to 10 drops of the blend to your diffuser, following the manufacturer's instructions. Label and store the remaining blend.
4. While the diffuser is running, enjoy the calm.

DIRECT INHALATION OPTION: If you would like to use this remedy on the go, use 8 to 10 drops of this blend in an aromatherapy inhaler. (See Antianxiety Inhaler on page 79 for instructions.) Breathe deeply from your inhaler to bring on a sense of focused, calm clarity anytime.

SELF-CARE BOOST: Making meditation a habit means you will be more likely to stick with your practice and enjoy all the mental and physical benefits that come with it. The easiest way to do this is to schedule a convenient time and place to meditate each day, even if you have only 5 minutes. Give it a try!

RAPID RECALL INHALER

This invigorating blend harnesses rosemary's renowned memory-boosting properties, along with invigorating peppermint, balancing marjoram, uplifting thyme, and a touch of sweet lavender. If you are feeling foggy and forgetful, reach for this inhaler to give your mind a quick performance boost. **DIRECT INHALATION, SAFE FOR AGES 10+, DO NOT USE IF PREGNANT OR BREASTFEEDING, DO NOT USE WITH BLOOD THINNERS**

3 drops rosemary essential oil

2 drops lavender essential oil

2 drops marjoram essential oil

2 drops peppermint essential oil

2 drops thyme essential oil

1. Put the essential oils in a small glass or ceramic bowl. Swirl the bowl around to blend the oils.

2. Put the cotton wick from the aromatherapy inhaler in the bowl and allow the wick to absorb the blend.

3. With a pair of tweezers, place the saturated wick into the aromatherapy inhaler and assemble. Snap or screw the cap into place. Affix a label to the inhaler.

4. Open the cap and inhale deeply through your nose as often as needed.

SELF-CARE BOOST: Research shows that our brains are constantly learning and changing, and we can improve our memory by putting it to work. Learn to play an instrument or take a little time to challenge yourself with brain teasers, sudoku, or crossword puzzles, which help keep certain areas of our brains active and flexible.

SPONGING UP / READY TO LEARN DIFFUSER BLEND

Whether you are studying, preparing for a presentation, or prepping for another task that requires memorization, this blend can help. With spearmint and lemon to stimulate cognition, rosemary to boost your memory, eucalyptus to enhance focus, and cypress to provide calm confidence, this diffuser blend is the ideal addition to a big day at work or school.

DIFFUSION, SAFE FOR AGES 2+, DO NOT USE IF PREGNANT OR BREASTFEEDING

---

10 drops rosemary essential oil

10 drops spearmint essential oil

8 drops eucalyptus essential oil

6 drops cypress essential oil

4 drops lemon essential oil

1. Put the essential oils in a small, dark-colored bottle. (If you are using a pipette to measure out the oils, use a new one for each essential oil—do not reuse.)

2. Cap the bottle tightly and swirl to blend the oils.

3. Add 8 to 10 drops of the blend to your diffuser, following the manufacturer's instructions. Label and store the remaining blend.

4. While the diffuser is running, start studying, preparing, or prepping.

DIRECT INHALATION OPTION: If you would like to use this remedy on the go, use 8 to 10 drops of this blend in an aromatherapy inhaler. (See Antianxiety Inhaler on page 79 for instructions.) Breathe deeply from your inhaler as often as needed to sharpen your memory and enhance cognition.

ACUPRESSURE TIP: The acupressure points on the top of your head are great for stimulating brain function. First, find DU20 by tracing a line from the highest point of your ears to the top of your head. Give that center spot a gentle 90-second massage. Now, begin making a circle around that point, about 1 inch out from DU20, and continue the acupressure massage, moving in a circle, for another 90 seconds. Now you are stimulating 4 points called "Si Shen Cong," which are known to enhance memory and concentration.

SELF-CARE BOOST: Exercise is great for your brain and can enhance your ability to retain information. If you want to learn something new and be able to recall it, try listening to the information while moving your body. For instance, listen to a podcast while using the elliptical.

REFRESH MY MEMORY DIFFUSER BLEND

Four of the most popular oils mingle in this simple blend to help you feel calm and alert. Basil is second only to rosemary for enhancing memory, and peppermint is close behind. This brightly scented duo helps focus your mind and sharpen your senses. Frankincense boosts mental clarity while aiding memory, and a touch of lavender alleviates any anxiety you are feeling about the task at hand. **DIFFUSION, SAFE FOR AGES 2+, DO NOT USE IF PREGNANT OR BREASTFEEDING**

4 drops peppermint
   essential oil
2 drops basil essential oil
2 drops frankincense
   essential oil
1 drop lavender essential oil

1. Put the essential oils in a small, dark-colored bottle. (If you are using a pipette to measure out the oils, use a new one for each essential oil—do not reuse.)

2. Cap the bottle tightly and swirl to blend the oils.

3. Add 8 to 10 drops of the blend to your diffuser, following the manufacturer's instructions. Label and store the remaining blend.

4. While the diffuser is running, start sorting through your memory bank.

DIRECT INHALATION OPTION: If you would like to use this remedy on the go, use 8 to 10 drops of this blend in an aromatherapy inhaler. (See Antianxiety Inhaler on page 79 for instructions.) Breathe deeply from your inhaler as often as needed to spark your memory.

SELF-CARE BOOST: Sleep and memory are interconnected. Memories consolidate while you are sound asleep, so to enhance your memory, be sure to enjoy as many quality z's as you can—ideally 7 to 8 hours per night.

RESTFUL SLUMBER BODY OIL

This deeply relaxing blend combines calming lavender and marjoram with soothing vetiver and a dash of lime to settle your nerves. When you are ready to dive under the covers, reach for this moisturizing body oil to promote total relaxation and sound sleep. **TOPICAL, SAFE FOR AGES 2+, DO NOT USE IF PREGNANT**

16 drops marjoram essential oil

16 drops lavender essential oil

4 drops vetiver essential oil

4 drops lime essential oil

4 ounces carrier oil

1. Put the essential oils in a 4-ounce, dark-colored bottle. Swirl to blend.

2. Add the carrier oil and cap the bottle tightly. Shake gently to mix.

3. For a relaxing bath, add 1 tablespoon of the oil to warm bathwater. To use as a moisturizer, rub about 1 teaspoon on your skin, using more or less as needed.

ACUPRESSURE TIP: Yin tang, located directly between the eyebrows, is one of the most calming acupressure points. Massage this point for up to 90 seconds as you begin to wind down for the night. Skip essential oils at this point to avoid getting anything in your eyes. Bonus: This point works great for kids!

SELF-CARE BOOST: Late-night TV watching and social media scrolling can be too stimulating for most people. Turn off the screens well before bedtime to get a better night's sleep.

SIMPLY SLEEP ROLL-ON

This ultra-simple blend pairs calming lavender with valerian, which is deeply comforting and wonderfully balancing. Together, these oils work as a natural relaxant that helps you find your way to dreamland. You will wake refreshed and ready to take on the day ahead. **TOPICAL, SAFE FOR AGES 2+, DO NOT USE IF PREGNANT, DO NOT USE WHILE DRIVING**

3 drops lavender
essential oil
3 drops valerian
essential oil
1¾ teaspoons jojoba oil

1. Using a fresh pipette for each oil, place the essential oils in a prelabeled 10-milliliter roller bottle. Add the jojoba oil.

2. Snap on the rollerball and screw on the cap. Shake until well-mixed.

3. Roll onto your wrists and other pulse points as needed.

SELF-CARE BOOST: Since caffeine stays in your system for several hours, it is important to limit intake during the day so that it does not hinder your ability to fall asleep. Try not to have any caffeine after lunch and consider reducing the amount of caffeine you consume overall.

PEACEFUL DREAMS DIFFUSER BLEND

Pacifying clary sage, tranquil ylang-ylang, and relaxing sage come together in a blend that is balanced by soothing sandalwood. This blend helps relieve tension and anxiety while promoting a sense of serenity. When your day has been hectic or emotions have run high, this blend will help soothe your busy mind so that you can sleep soundly. **DIFFUSION, SAFE FOR AGES 2+, DO NOT USE IF PREGNANT OR BREASTFEEDING**

15 drops clary sage essential oil
15 drops sandalwood essential oil
15 drops ylang-ylang essential oil
10 drops sage essential oil

1. Put the essential oils in a small, dark-colored bottle. (If you are using a pipette to measure out the oils, use a new one for each essential oil—do not reuse.)

2. Cap the bottle tightly and swirl to blend the oils.

3. Add 8 to 10 drops of the blend to your diffuser, following the manufacturer's instructions. Label and store the remaining blend.

4. While the diffuser is running, allow yourself to drift off to sleep.

SELF-CARE BOOST: Regulating your body's clock by setting a regular bedtime and wake-up time can set the stage for regular restful sleep. Staying up too late or sleeping in all day on weekends can also impact your sleep during the week. If you have difficulty sleeping, set a schedule and stick to it, even on weekends.

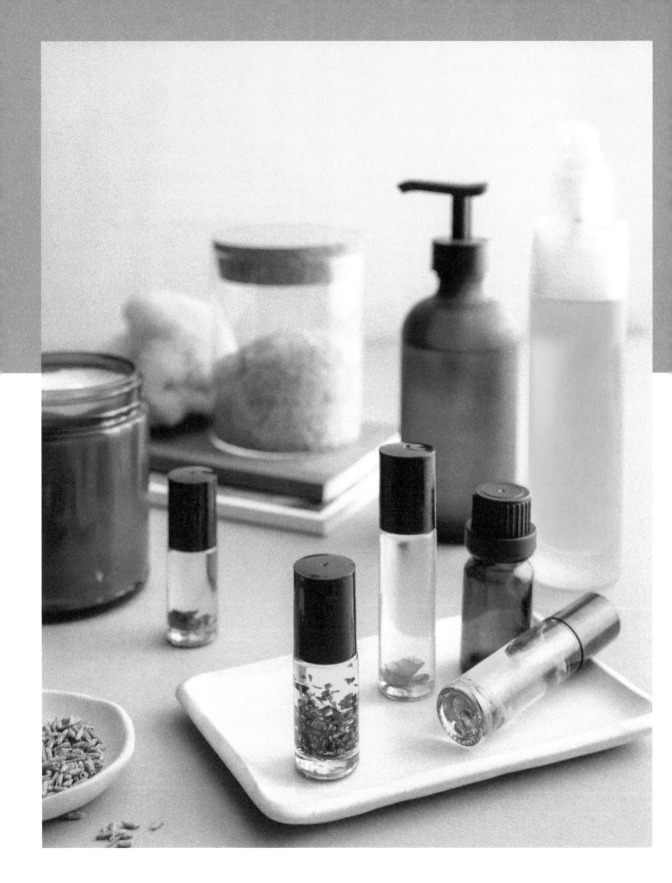

07

Physical Well-Being

Whether you find yourself dealing with a common skin problem such as acne or facing another issue like muscle aches, a sore throat, or even an itchy case of athlete's foot, aromatherapy can help. The remedies in this chapter are mostly applied topically, making use of essential oils such as tea tree and lavender for their antibacterial, antifungal, and antiviral properties, as well as favorites like helichrysum and frankincense, valued for their ability to aid in skin regeneration while promoting healing from within. Of course, you will find many others here, too! When you are searching for easy ways to look and feel your best, consider reaching for your essential oils. You may be astonished at the difference they can make in your physical well-being.

ANTIACNE SCRUB

This invigorating scrub replaces harsh chemicals with anti-inflammatory yarrow, antiseptic tea tree, and healing lavender to gently unclog pores and kill bacteria while giving skin a fresh, glowing appearance. Bentonite clay reduces oil production and helps unclog pores, whereas oat flour gently exfoliates. Use this scrub alone or pair it with traditional acne products to give pimples and blackheads a one-two punch. **TOPICAL, SAFE FOR AGES 10+, DO NOT USE IF PREGNANT, DO NOT USE WITH DRUGS METABOLIZED BY CYP2D6**

6 tablespoons oat flour

4 tablespoons bentonite clay

2 tablespoons aluminum-free baking soda

6 tablespoons jojoba oil or liquid coconut oil

10 drops lavender essential oil

10 drops rose hip oil (optional)

10 drops tea tree essential oil

10 drops yarrow essential oil

1. In an 8-ounce glass jar, combine the oat flour, bentonite clay, and baking soda. Use a thin utensil to mix completely.

2. Add the remaining ingredients. Stir again until combined.

3. Cap tightly. Label the jar and store the scrub in a cool, dark place for up to 6 months.

4. To use, apply 1 teaspoon of the facial scrub to your face and other body parts affected by acne. Massage in gentle circular motions for at least 30 seconds.

5. After massaging for at least 30 seconds, use a soft wet cloth to rinse away the scrub. Follow up with toner and moisturizer, if you like.

6. Repeat 3 or 4 times weekly.

TECHNIQUE TIP: For a thinner consistency, add up to 1 tablespoon more of whichever carrier oil you are using.

SELF-CARE BOOST: In many cases, acne results from stress, digestive issues or food sensitivities, environmental factors, products we use on our skin, and more. While treating the problem can help you look and feel better, it is vital to uncover the root cause and address it. Your skin and your self-esteem will benefit.

PATCHOULI-CHAMOMILE SUGAR SCRUB

Cleanse and exfoliate in one quick step with this comforting sugar scrub. Patchouli and Roman chamomile essential oils nourish and balance the skin and add a lovely scent to your daily routine. **TOPICAL, SAFE FOR AGES 12+**

8 drops patchouli essential oil

4 drops Roman chamomile essential oil

½ cup sweet almond oil

½ cup sugar

1. In a jar with a tight-fitting lid, combine the patchouli and Roman chamomile essential oils. Let the blend rest for at least 1 hour.

2. Using a thin utensil such as a fork or butter knife, stir in the almond oil and sugar to blend completely.

3. Dampen your face with warm water. With your fingertips, apply about ½ teaspoon of the sugar scrub to your face. Using gentle circular motions, cleanse your entire face.

4. Rinse your face thoroughly with warm water and pat it dry with a soft towel. Repeat daily.

5. Keep the scrub in a convenient location away from heat.

TECHNIQUE TIP: This sugar scrub is not a treat just for your face—it will smooth and moisturize your entire body. Use it in the shower for softly scented skin that looks and feels fantastic.

NOURISHING ROSE ANTIAGING SERUM

Soothe and soften skin while gently combating wrinkles with this blend of regenerative, astringent, and anti-inflammatory essential oils. Together, rose, helichrysum, frankincense, and rose geranium essential oils heal, nurture, and tighten your skin from the inside out. If you do not have jojoba, you can use liquid coconut oil instead, which is also an excellent choice. **TOPICAL, SAFE FOR AGES 2+**

1 (1-ounce) bottle jojoba oil with a pump or dropper top

18 drops rose essential oil (optional)

18 drops rose geranium essential oil

9 drops frankincense essential oil

9 drops helichrysum essential oil

1. Transfer 54 drops of the jojoba oil from the bottle to a separate container, using the dropper top or pipette. Set aside for future use.

2. Add the essential oils to the bottle of remaining jojoba oil. Cap tightly and shake for about 10 seconds to blend. Affix a label and store in the refrigerator for up to 6 months.

3. Apply just 2 or 3 drops to your freshly washed face, using a little more or less of the serum as needed. Repeat twice daily as part of your regular skincare regimen.

SELF-CARE BOOST: Want dewy, youthful skin? Drink up! When the skin is dehydrated, it shows age faster, so make sure you are drinking 8 to 10 glasses of water a day. Your skin will thank you.

NATURAL FRESHNESS MOUTH RINSE

With antibacterial lemon and thyme, plus refreshing spearmint to leave breath smelling its best, this natural mouthwash includes a touch of liquid stevia for chemical-free sweetness. Used as part of your daily oral health routine, this rinse easily replaces expensive, chemical-laden commercial options. Reach for it anytime your mouth is feeling less than fresh. **TOPICAL, SAFE FOR AGES 12+, DO NOT USE WITH BLOOD THINNERS**

1 tablespoon witch hazel, preferably alcohol-free
1 teaspoon liquid coconut oil
8 drops spearmint essential oil
5 drops thyme essential oil
4 drops lemon essential oil
3 cups distilled water
8 drops liquid stevia (optional)
1 tablespoon aluminum-free baking soda

1. In a 2-quart mason jar or glass container with a tight-fitting lid, combine the witch hazel, coconut oil, and essential oils. Stir well.

2. Add the water, stevia (if using), and the baking soda. Cap the jar tightly and shake it until the baking soda has completely dissolved.

3. Affix a label to the jar and store it in the refrigerator for up to 4 weeks.

4. To use, swish 1 tablespoon of the rinse around in your mouth after brushing your teeth; after a few moments, spit it out. Use after both morning and night brushings.

SELF-CARE BOOST: If you are paying close attention to oral hygiene and you are still suffering from bad breath, talk with your health-care practitioner about the issue; halitosis (bad breath) can be a symptom of an underlying condition.

FIRST-AID SALVE FOR BLISTERS AND MORE

Try this comforting first-aid remedy to help a blister heal faster while easing some of the discomfort. Virgin coconut oil and lavender offer pain relief as well as antibacterial action, whereas soothing Roman chamomile helps ease the swelling. This remedy is also good for minor wounds, razor burns, stings, cuts, and scrapes. However, be sure to see your health-care practitioner for puncture wounds, serious cuts, and other injuries that might need medical attention beyond at-home first aid. **TOPICAL, SAFE FOR AGES 2+, DO NOT USE IF PREGNANT**

2 tablespoons beeswax pastilles or grated beeswax

2 tablespoons virgin coconut oil

1 tablespoon shea butter or cocoa butter

¼ cup jojoba oil

6 drops Roman chamomile essential oil

3 drops lavender essential oil

1. In a heat-safe glass measuring cup with a handle or in a double boiler, melt the beeswax over barely simmering water over medium-low heat; it should take about 10 to 15 minutes. (To avoid a grainy product, melt the beeswax completely.)

2. Remove the glass cup or the upper section of the double boiler from the heat and immediately add the premeasured coconut oil, butter, and jojoba oil to the melted beeswax. (Do not allow the beeswax to harden.)

3. Allow the blend to cool for 1 to 2 minutes and then add the essential oils. Use a thin utensil to thoroughly blend the salve.

   Pour the salve while it is still soft into an 8-ounce jar with a tight-fitting lid. (If you prefer to keep the balm in multiple locations, you can pour it into several smaller containers that have caps.)

4. Allow the salve to cool completely before capping and affixing a label.

5. Apply a pea-size amount of the salve to the blister after bathing or showering and before bedtime, rubbing gently to smooth the blend over your skin. Cover with a bandage if needed. For larger areas, use more salve.

SELF-CARE BOOST: If your blister was caused by shoes, avoid shoes that aggravate the area and use a blister cushion to protect the area while it heals. These cushions can also help prevent new blisters from forming. If you have been getting lots of blisters on your feet, take a look at your shoes to see if they are to blame—they might be too big or too small.

BACK TO BALANCE
BATH SALTS

This blend combines four of the most effective diuretic oils with the aim of reducing fluid accumulation under the skin. Fresh-scented lemon and grapefruit add energizing, euphoric notes whereas fennel and rosemary provide warm herbal tones. Epsom salts help you unwind and avocado oil leaves your skin feeling soft. **TOPICAL, SAFE FOR AGES 5+, DO NOT USE WITH BLOOD THINNERS, NOT RECOMMENDED FOR THOSE WITH ENDOME-TRIOSIS OR AN ESTROGEN-DEPENDENT CANCER**

8 drops grapefruit
essential oil

8 drops lemon
essential oil

8 drops fennel
essential oil

4 drops rosemary
essential oil

1 tablespoon avocado oil

4 cups Epsom salts

1. In a large mixing bowl, combine the essential oils and the avocado oil.

2. Add the Epsom salts and stir the mixture with a metal utensil until thoroughly combined.

3. Using a large spoon, transfer the bath salts to a quart-size jar with a tight-fitting lid. Affix a label and store the jar in a cool, dark place for up to 2 months.

4. Use about ½ cup of bath salts in a warm bath, stirring it into the water with your hand. Relax in the tub for at least 15 minutes. Repeat daily or as often as needed to encourage your body to release retained water.

TECHNIQUE TIP: Omit the rosemary essential oil if you plan to go to bed immediately following the bath.

SELF-CARE BOOST: If you are not certain what is causing your body to retain water, it is a good idea to check in with your health-care practitioner. Frequent or severe water retention can be a symptom of an underlying condition.

LAVENDER-LEMONGRASS DEODORANT SPRAY

Lemongrass is such an effective deodorizer that it's a top ingredient in some bestselling natural deodorant brands. Natural deodorants made with essential oils won't keep you from sweating, but they do kill bacteria that cause body odor—plus, they'll keep you smelling nice. **TOPICAL, SAFE FOR AGES 12+**

30 drops lavender
    essential oil
30 drops lemongrass
    essential oil
⅛ teaspoon unprocessed
    sea salt or fine
    Himalayan salt
6 tablespoons alcohol-free
    witch hazel
8 ounces magnesium oil

1. In a glass bottle fitted with a spray top, combine the lavender and lemongrass essential oils. Let them rest for at least 1 hour.

2. Add the salt and swirl to combine.

3. Add the witch hazel and magnesium oil, cap the bottle, and shake well to combine. Shake again before each use.

4. Apply 1 or 2 spritzes to each underarm. Repeat as needed.

5. Keep the deodorant in a cool, dry place between uses.

TECHNIQUE TIP: You can easily make your own signature deodorant by substituting your favorite essential oils for the ones called for here.

SOOTHING BRUISE BALM

With arnica cream as a carrier, this blend relieves pain from deep bruising while encouraging better circulation and promoting faster healing. Cypress penetrates deeply into tissue to calm inflammation, whereas helichrysum offers pain-relieving, regenerative, and anti-inflammatory properties. Hyssop adds a comforting note to the blend while working as an antiseptic. This calming, balancing blend isn't just good for bruises; it is also a soothing balm for overworked muscles. **TOPICAL, SAFE FOR AGES 2+, DO NOT USE IF PREGNANT OR BREASTFEEDING**

---

2 ounces arnica cream
18 drops cypress
    essential oil
18 drops hyssop
    essential oil
18 drops helichrysum
    essential oil

1. Put the arnica cream in a small glass or metal bowl. Add the essential oils and, using a thin utensil, stir until completely blended.

2. Transfer the finished balm to a small glass jar with a tight-fitting lid and cap tightly. Affix a label and store it in a cool, dark place for up to 6 months.

3. Apply a pea-size amount of the balm to your bruise once or twice daily. Use a little more or less as needed to cover the bruised area. Repeat daily until the bruise fades.

SELF-CARE BOOST: If you bruise easily, talk with your health-care practitioner about whether supplemental vitamin C and vitamin K might help make you less prone to bruising. Vitamin C strengthens the walls of your red blood cells and vitamin K helps improve clotting, which can reduce the size of a bruise.

LAVENDER MOISTURIZING LIP BALM

This healing blend includes helichrysum for its regenerative, anti-inflammatory, and pain-relieving attributes, plus clary sage and lavender to increase the soothing effect while adding a touch of antibacterial potency. Coconut oil and cocoa butter add moisture, and beeswax imparts a firmness that helps seal in moisture while healing painful cracks. This balm can be placed in a few small jars or tins or poured into lip balm tubes. **TOPICAL, SAFE FOR AGES 6+, DO NOT USE IF PREGNANT**

1 tablespoon beeswax pastilles

1 tablespoon virgin coconut oil

1 tablespoon cocoa butter

3 drops helichrysum essential oil

2 drops clary sage essential oil

1 drop lavender essential oil

1. In a double boiler, melt the beeswax over barely simmering water; it should take about 10 to 15 minutes. (To avoid a grainy product, melt the beeswax completely.)

2. Remove the upper section of the double boiler from the heat, and immediately add the coconut oil and cocoa butter to the melted beeswax. (Do not allow the beeswax to harden.)

3. Allow this base to cool for 1 to 2 minutes and then add the essential oils. Use a thin utensil to thoroughly blend the balm.

4. While the balm is still soft, use a funnel to pour it into lip balm tubes or other containers. Allow it to cool completely before capping and affixing a label.

5. Use as needed to soothe chapped lips.

TECHNIQUE TIP: If you want to use lip balm tubes, you will need about 7 of them for this recipe. You will also need a way to keep them upright when you fill them. While you can buy a tool just for this, if you do not want to make the investment, you can fill a shallow dish with uncooked rice and position the empty tubes between the grains.

SELF-CARE BOOST: Dry, air-conditioned or heated indoor air and arid outdoor conditions make your lips prone to chapping and licking them makes matters worse. Keep your lips protected with a layer of comforting balm or your favorite lipstick and you will be less likely to find yourself dealing with severe chapping.

BREATHE EASY STEAM INHALATION

This inhalation makes the most of eucalyptus, which is such a potent decongestant that it is used in a number of commercial preparations. Sage adds antibacterial and anti-inflammatory properties while easing the discomfort that can accompany congestion. Spearmint is another decongestant, and it adds a refreshing note that keeps the blend from smelling overly medicinal. **DIRECT INHALATION, SAFE FOR AGES 10+, DO NOT USE IF PREGNANT OR BREASTFEEDING**

3 drops eucalyptus
   essential oil
2 drops sage essential oil
1 drop spearmint
   essential oil

1. Fill a large pot with 1 inch of water. On the stovetop, bring the water to a boil. Alternatively, fill a large glass bowl with about 1 inch of water and bring it to a boil in the microwave.

2. Spread out a large bath towel on your tabletop. Have a box of tissues nearby.

3. Carefully set the pot or bowl of steaming water on the towel and add the essential oils.

4. Sit at the table in front of the pot and drape a second bath towel over your head and the pot, creating a tent that traps the steam. Breathe deeply.

5. If you feel too hot or need to blow your nose, take breaks from the steam. Continue for 10 minutes, or until the water cools and stops steaming.

6. Repeat once or twice daily when congestion is an issue.

DIRECT INHALATION OR DIFFUSION OPTIONS: If you do not have time for a steam, you can use this blend in an aromatherapy inhaler. (See Antianxiety Inhaler on page 79 for instructions.) You can also use this blend in your diffuser, following the manufacturer's instructions. These methods will not be quite as powerful as steam inhalation, but you will still likely feel less congested with this remedy on hand.

ACUPRESSURE TIP: If you are suffering from sinus congestion, try this acupressure combo to help open up your sinuses. Gently massage the following points for 90 seconds: Yin tang (located between the eyebrows) and Large Intestine 20 (located on each side of the nostrils where the nose meets the groove of the smile line).

SELF-CARE BOOST: The steam from a hot shower can help clear congestion. Any one of the oils in this remedy can be used to help you breathe a little easier. Just add 3 drops of the essential oil to a washcloth, place it on the shower floor, and enjoy your shower as usual.

FLAKE-FREE SHAMPOO AND CONDITIONER

With your favorite unscented shampoo and conditioner as a convenient base, this blend includes antifungal tea tree and lemongrass oils along with antibacterial thyme. These essential oils also offer pain-relieving properties that can help soothe the itch that accompanies dandruff. A teaspoon of your favorite carrier oil adds just a touch of extra moisture to each remedy. **TOPICAL, SAFE FOR AGES 2+, DO NOT USE IF PREGNANT OR BREASTFEEDING, DO NOT USE WITH BLOOD THINNERS, DO NOT USE WITH DRUGS METABOLIZED BY CYP2B6**

For the shampoo

30 drops lemongrass essential oil
20 drops thyme essential oil
20 drops tea tree essential oil
1 teaspoon jojoba or another carrier oil
1 cup unscented shampoo

For the conditioner

30 drops lemongrass essential oil
20 drops thyme essential oil
20 drops tea tree essential oil
10 drops lavender essential oil (optional)
1 teaspoon jojoba or another carrier oil
1 cup unscented conditioner

1. Put the essential oils for the shampoo in a medium bowl. Add the carrier oil and stir to combine. Slowly add the unscented shampoo and mix until thoroughly blended.

2. Using a funnel, transfer the shampoo to a shatterproof 8-ounce bottle approved for use with essential oils.

3. Put the essential oils for the conditioner in a second bowl. Add the carrier oil and stir to combine. Slowly add the unscented conditioner and mix until thoroughly blended.

4. With a clean funnel, transfer the conditioner to a second 8-ounce bottle.

5. Label the bottles, cap them tightly, and store them in the shower. Shampoo and condition your hair once daily to help keep dandruff under control.

SELF-CARE BOOST: Apple cider vinegar kills fungus, including the kind that commonly contributes to dandruff. Mix equal parts of water and apple cider vinegar in a plastic squeeze bottle with an applicator tip and apply it to your entire scalp. Let it sit for 5 minutes and then rinse it out before finishing with shampoo and conditioner. This helps speed the healing process and dramatically eases itching. Repeat this treatment for 5 to 7 days for best results.

MOISTURIZING HAIR MASK

This conditioning hair mask includes uplifting bergamot and soothing lavender in addition to rosemary, which finds its way into many commercial products. This blend promotes healthy circulation in your scalp and the soothing oils penetrate thirsty strands, leaving hair feeling silky-soft once the treatment has been completed. **TOPICAL, SAFE FOR AGES 2+**

½ cup virgin coconut oil

¼ cup jojoba oil or other carrier oil

8 drops bergamot essential oil

6 drops rosemary essential oil

4 drops lavender essential oil

1. In a mixing bowl, combine all the ingredients.

2. Whip the blend with an electric mixer on medium-to-high speed for about 5 minutes, or until smooth and creamy.

3. With a spatula or spoon, transfer the finished hair mask to a jar. Label the jar and cap it tightly. Store the mask in the refrigerator between uses.

4. Apply 1 tablespoon of the hair mask to clean, dry hair, using more or less as needed depending on its length. Comb the mask through the strands so that they are all coated.

5. You can cover your hair with a towel or protective cap to protect your clothing or furniture, if you would like. Set a timer for 15 minutes and relax while the blend does its work.

6. When the timer goes off, wash your hair 2 or 3 times as needed to remove the excess oil. Condition, dry, and style as usual. Enjoy your hair mask at least once a week or even more often if your hair can really use it.

SELF-CARE BOOST: If you can stand it, use cool water rather than hot water to rinse out your shampoo and conditioner. Hot water strips the moisture from hair while cold water helps the hair's cuticles lie flat, sealing moisture inside and promoting a shiny appearance and silky feel.

DEEP MOISTURE BODY OIL

Rich avocado oil penetrates deeply without leaving a greasy film behind. This body oil contains helichrysum to aid in regeneration while providing anti-inflammatory action, myrrh for its peaceful aroma and detoxifying effect, and patchouli, which adds a wonderful note of warmth to the blend. **TOPICAL, SAFE FOR AGES 2+, DO NOT USE IF PREGNANT OR BREASTFEEDING, DO NOT USE WITH BLOOD THINNERS**

12 drops sandalwood essential oil

12 drops patchouli essential oil

10 drops myrrh essential oil

10 drops helichrysum essential oil

7½ ounces avocado oil

1 teaspoon vitamin E oil (optional)

1. Put the essential oils in an 8-ounce bottle with a tight-fitting lid or pump top. Swirl for about 5 seconds to blend.

2. Add the avocado oil and the vitamin E oil, if using. Cap tightly and then shake well to combine thoroughly. Label the bottle and store it in a cool, dark place for up to 6 months.

3. Apply about 1 teaspoon of moisturizing oil to your entire body, using more or less as needed to cover. This body oil is best enjoyed after your daily bath or shower.

SELF-CARE BOOST: Arid indoor air can make dry skin even worse. If this is an issue for you, consider running a humidifier in your home to keep the air moist and your skin hydrated.

DEODORIZING FOOT SPRAY

This refreshing spray combines energizing tea tree with healing sage and soothing lavender, creating a wonderful fragrance that makes this quick self-care ritual feel like a mini-spa treatment. These essential oils are also excellent for their antibacterial and antifungal properties, effectively eliminating the microbes that cause stinky feet. **TOPICAL, SAFE FOR AGES 2+, DO NOT USE IF PREGNANT OR BREASTFEEDING**

6 drops tea tree
   essential oil
4 drops sage essential oil
2 drops lavender
   essential oil
½ cup witch hazel

1. Combine the essential oils in a 4-ounce bottle that can be fitted with a spray top. Swirl for about 5 seconds to blend.

2. Add the witch hazel. Cap the bottle and shake well. Affix a label. (The witch hazel should completely emulsify the essential oils; if there is a layer of essential oil floating on top of the witch hazel, shake before each use.)

3. Pump 2 or 3 spritzes of spray onto your clean, dry feet, ensuring that you get it between your toes. Let your feet dry completely before putting on socks and shoes. Repeat daily as needed.

SELF-CARE BOOST: Moisture trapped in shoes contributes to foot odor, so keep your shoes dry. If your shoes are smelly, sprinkle the insides with a blend made from ½ cup baking soda and 10 drops tea tree oil mixed together. Sprinkle ½ teaspoon into each shoe and allow it to sit. Shake out any excess powder before you put the shoes back on.

SOOTHING HEADACHE ROLL-ON

In this roll-on, calming cedarwood blends with marjoram, peppermint, eucalyptus, and lavender. These four oils are well known for their pain-relieving properties. Both soothing and energizing, this blend helps take your mind off your headache while encouraging your whole body to relax. **TOPICAL, SAFE FOR AGES 2+, DO NOT USE IF PREGNANT OR BREASTFEEDING**

3 drops peppermint essential oil

2 drops cedarwood essential oil

2 drops eucalyptus essential oil

2 drops lavender essential oil

2 drops marjoram essential oil

1¾ teaspoons jojoba oil

1. Using a fresh pipette for each oil, place the essential oils in a prelabeled 10-milliliter roller bottle. Add the jojoba oil.

2. Snap on the rollerball and screw on the cap. Shake until well-mixed.

3. Roll onto your temples and the back of your neck as needed. Massage your head while taking deep, relaxing breaths for a minute or so to treat yourself.

SELF-CARE BOOST: Many headaches originate from tight, tense muscles in the neck that radiate tension up into the tiny muscles of the scalp and face. Some common causes of neck tension include stress, poor posture, and staying in one position for long periods (perhaps while working on computers or looking at those small phone and tablet screens). If you sit at a desk for several hours at a time, consider taking a few minutes to stretch your neck, back, and shoulders every hour. Moving can help you feel better now and it helps prevent similar headaches in the future.

TUMMY TAMER ROLL-ON

Along with comforting fennel, invigorating peppermint, and reassuring coriander to stimulate the digestive tract, this blend includes Roman chamomile to combat the inflammation that often accompanies indigestion. Reach for this roll-on when your digestive tract feels uncomfortable. Whether the trouble is gas and bloating, sluggish digestion, nausea, or another form of upset, this blend can help you feel better. **TOPICAL, SAFE FOR AGES 6+, DO NOT USE IF PREGNANT OR BREASTFEEDING, DO NOT USE WITH BLOOD THINNERS, DO NOT USE IF YOU HAVE ENDOMETRIOSIS OR AN ESTROGEN-DEPENDENT CANCER**

9 drops fennel essential oil

8 drops Roman chamomile essential oil

6 drops coriander essential oil

5 drops peppermint essential oil

1¾ teaspoons jojoba oil

1. Using a fresh pipette for each oil, put the essential oils in a prelabeled 10-milliliter roller bottle. Add the jojoba oil.

2. Snap on the rollerball and screw on the cap. Shake until well-mixed.

3. Roll this blend onto your abdomen and massage it in with your fingers, preferably while relaxing. Begin your abdominal massage at the belly button and work your way outward in a clockwise direction, using gentle pressure. Use light pressure at first, and then gradually increase it but do not press so hard that you make your discomfort worse. Make at least 10 rotations and continue for a longer period if you have time. Repeat as needed.

ACUPRESSURE TIP: Ren 12 (located midway between your belly button and the bottom edge of your sternum) can help harmonize the abdomen. Use the roll-on and massage the blend into this point, and you should feel relief in no time.

SELF-CARE BOOST: When indigestion comes calling, have a cup of tea to soothe the upset. Great choices for digestive relief include peppermint tea and ginger tea.

IN THE MOOD LINEN SPRAY

This delightfully exotic, lightly spicy blend includes a trio of natural aphrodisiacs—ginger, jasmine, and ylang-ylang. Wonderful for creating a romantic atmosphere and stimulating pleasure centers in the brain, these essential oils are also among the most relaxing. Because tension, stress, and anxiety often contribute to low libido, this blend is formulated to address them while helping you get in the mood. If this blend seems a little too heavy for you, try adding 4 to 8 drops sweet orange to lighten it just a touch. **ATMOSPHERIC DIFFUSION, SAFE FOR AGES 2+**

16 drops ginger essential oil
8 drops jasmine essential oil (optional)
8 drops ylang-ylang essential oil
1 cup unflavored vodka

1. Put the essential oils in an 8-ounce bottle that can be fitted with a spray top and swirl for about 5 seconds to blend.

2. Add the vodka. Cap the bottle and shake well to blend completely. Add a label and allow the blend to rest for 1 or 2 days to give the fragrance an opportunity to develop.

3. Spritz your linens as often as you like to give your entire bed a pleasing, romantic fragrance. You can use this blend on other textiles, too: Try it on curtains and carpets to give your entire bedroom a welcoming, sensual atmosphere.

SELF-CARE BOOST: Wondering where your sex drive went? Two of the biggest culprits are high stress and hormonal imbalances. Managing stress can make a huge difference, but if that does not help you get your game back, check in with your doctor to have hormone labs run.

CRAMPS BEGONE MASSAGE OIL

Get relief from the pain of menstrual cramps with this relaxing blend. Formulated with clary sage and fennel to encourage smooth muscle tissue to relax, it includes rose geranium to ease stress while contributing a light floral note to the blend. Rose geranium and fennel are diuretics, so this blend can help relieve bloating and water retention that coincide with your cycle. **TOPICAL, SAFE FOR AGES 5+, DO NOT USE IF PREGNANT OR BREASTFEEDING, NOT RECOMMENDED FOR USE IF YOU HAVE ENDOMETRIOSIS OR AN ESTROGEN-DEPENDENT CANCER**

16 drops clary sage essential oil
8 drops fennel essential oil
8 drops rose geranium essential oil
4 ounces carrier oil

1. Put the essential oils in a 4-ounce, dark-colored bottle. Swirl to blend.

2. Add the carrier oil and cap the bottle tightly. Shake gently to mix.

3. For a soothing massage, apply about ¼ teaspoon to your lower abdomen, using more or less as needed. While relaxing in a reclined position, move your fingertips in small circles, focusing on the area where the discomfort is most intense. Gradually make your circles larger until you are massaging the entire lower abdomen. Continue this comforting massage for about 3 to 5 minutes.

BATH OPTION: For a relaxing bath, add 1 tablespoon of this blend to warm bathwater, along with ½ cup to 1 cup Epsom salts, if you would like, for additional relief.

SELF-CARE BOOST: When you start to feel cramps coming on, relax with a heating pad on your lower back for 10 minutes. Then, switch the heating pad to the front over your lower abdomen for another 10 minutes. Alternate again for as long as it feels good to you, but for safety, be sure that your heating pad is turned off before you go to sleep.

PAIN AWAY ROLL-ON

This complex blend brings 5 pain-relieving essential oils together. With a hint of bracing peppermint, energizing basil, soothing Roman chamomile, calming marjoram, and a touch of helichrysum and lavender for added anti-inflammatory action, this combo goes deep into muscles to soothe tension. **TOPICAL, SAFE FOR AGES 6+, DO NOT USE IF PREGNANT OR BREASTFEEDING**

---

3 drops peppermint essential oil

3 drops basil essential oil

2 drops marjoram essential oil

1 drop helichrysum essential oil

1 drop lavender essential oil

1 drop Roman chamomile essential oil

1¾ teaspoons jojoba oil

1. Using a fresh pipette for each oil, put the essential oils in a prelabeled 10-milliliter roller bottle. Add the jojoba oil.

2. Snap on the rollerball and screw on the cap. Shake until well-mixed.

3. Apply the blend to the temples, forehead, and base of the skull, massaging in small circles while breathing deeply and focusing on relaxation. Take time out for some simple stretches or a quick walk around the block to enhance circulation and reduce muscle tension.

ACUPRESSURE TIP: Large Intestine 4 (located on the backside of the hand, on the fleshy mound between the thumb and index finger) is known as the "command point of the face." Use moderate pressure to stimulate this point for up to 90 seconds to help kick the migraine.

SELF-CARE BOOST: Reach for this helpful roll-on at the first hint of a migraine and feel free to pair it with other remedies. If you take migraine medicine, double-check with your health-care practitioner to ensure that this blend will not interact with prescribed pharmaceuticals.

DEEP RELIEF MASSAGE OIL

The anti-inflammatory and pain-relieving properties of lavender, yarrow, rosemary, peppermint, and ginger combine in this helpful blend, which is ideal for aches and pains. If you are suffering from muscle spasms, this blend can help relax them as well. **TOPICAL, SAFE FOR AGES 6+, DO NOT USE IF PREGNANT OR BREASTFEEDING, DO NOT USE WITH DRUGS METABOLIZED BY CYP2D6**

16 drops yarrow essential oil

8 drops lavender essential oil

4 drops rosemary essential oil

4 drops peppermint essential oil

2 drops ginger essential oil

4 ounces carrier oil

1. Put the essential oils in a 4-ounce, dark-colored bottle. Swirl to blend.

2. Add the carrier oil and cap the bottle tightly. Shake gently to mix.

3. For a soothing massage, apply about ¼ teaspoon to the affected area, using a little more or less as needed. Spend at least 2 to 3 minutes gently massaging in circular motions. Repeat as needed.

BATH OPTION: For a relaxing bath, add 1 tablespoon of this blend to warm bathwater, along with ½ cup to 1 cup Epsom salts, if desired, for additional relief. Omit the ginger essential oil if you are using this blend in your bath.

ACUPRESSURE TIP: Spleen 21 (located on the side of the ribs below the armpit) is a great point for all-over body pain. Stimulate this point by using moderate pressure for up to 90 seconds. Bonus points if you use Deep Relief Massage Oil!

SELF-CARE BOOST: In herbal form, valerian is an excellent natural remedy for muscle pain. Consider taking a valerian supplement or drinking an herbal tea that includes valerian if muscle pain keeps you from relaxing or sleeping at night.

ANTINAUSEA INHALER

With a trio of antinausea essential oils, including peppermint, ginger, and lemongrass, this blend can short-circuit the messages between the brain and your stomach, easing the sickening sensations. This inhaler can be a lifesaver if you suffer from motion sickness or a nervous stomach. If you are looking for a way to deal with the nausea associated with morning sickness, skip the peppermint, which is not recommended during pregnancy, and create the roll-on with 6 drops ginger and 6 drops lemongrass, or simply inhale the ginger on its own. **DIRECT INHALATION, SAFE FOR AGES 6+**

6 drops peppermint essential oil

3 drops ginger essential oil

3 drops lemongrass essential oil

1. Put the essential oils in a small glass or ceramic bowl. Swirl the bowl around to blend the oils.

2. Put the cotton wick from the aromatherapy inhaler in the bowl and allow the wick to absorb the blend.

3. With a pair of tweezers, place the saturated wick into the aromatherapy inhaler and assemble. Snap or screw the cap into place. Affix a label to the inhaler.

4. Open the cap and inhale deeply through your nose as often as needed to reduce nausea.

ACUPRESSURE TIP: Pericardium 6 (located on the inner wrist) is known for its ability to settle nausea (which is why seasickness bands apply pressure there). To ease nausea, apply moderate pressure on this point for up to 90 seconds.

SELF-CARE BOOST: Next time you feel your stomach turning, have a soothing cup of chamomile tea or peppermint tea. Both herbs are renowned for their ability to ease nausea.

BALANCING SHAMPOO AND CONDITIONER

Both yarrow and rosemary are traditional treatments for balancing oily hair and both are found in commercial products designed to eliminate excess oil while leaving hair soft, shiny, and full. These essential oils give a fresh, herbal scent to this DIY shampoo and conditioner duo. If you find the fragrance too sharp, add up to 10 drops lavender to each bowl while blending the oils. **TOPICAL, SAFE FOR AGES 10+, DO NOT USE WITH DRUGS METABOLIZED BY CYP2D6**

For the shampoo

20 drops rosemary
    essential oil
20 drops yarrow
    essential oil
¼ teaspoon jojoba or
    another carrier oil
1 cup unscented shampoo

For the conditioner

20 drops rosemary
    essential oil
20 drops yarrow
    essential oil
¼ teaspoon jojoba or
    another carrier oil
1 cup unscented
    conditioner

1. Put the essential oils for the shampoo in a medium bowl. Add the carrier oil and stir to combine. Slowly add the unscented shampoo and mix until thoroughly blended.

2. Using a funnel, transfer the shampoo to a shatterproof 8-ounce bottle approved for use with essential oils.

3. Put the essential oils for the conditioner in a second bowl. Add the carrier oil and stir to combine. Slowly add the unscented conditioner and mix until thoroughly blended.

4. With a clean funnel, transfer the conditioner to a second 8-ounce bottle.

5. Label the bottles, cap them tightly, and store them in the shower. Shampoo and condition your hair once daily to balance oil production and keep your hair looking its best.

SELF-CARE BOOST: Scrubbing too hard can overstimulate the oil glands in your scalp and increase sebum production. Be sure to scrub gently and rinse thoroughly. When conditioning, focus on the ends of your hair and try not to get too much product on your scalp since its residue can make your hair look and feel greasy.

DETOXIFYING HAIR AND SCALP MUD MASK

If your scalp is more oily than usual, it's probably time for an exfoliation. It's a good idea to exfoliate your hair and scalp once a month to help regulate oil production and improve luster. **TOPICAL, SAFE FOR AGES 2+ YEARS**

¾ cup bentonite clay
1 tablespoon hemp seed oil
2 drops frankincense essential oil
2 drops sweet marjoram essential oil

1. In a medium bowl, thoroughly mix the bentonite clay, hemp seed oil, and essential oils.

2. Mix in water one tablespoon at a time, until the blend is spreadable but not drippy.

3. Apply mixture to hair, cover with a shower cap to retain heat, and let stand for 15 minutes to an hour.

4. Rinse completely and follow with an apple cider vinegar hair rinse.

TECHNIQUE TIP: This mud mask dries out hair the longer you leave it on, so it helps to spritz your hair with filtered water every so often.

REFRESHING OIL PULL BLEND

This invigorating blend includes antibacterial essential oils that get rid of germs that contribute to bad breath, plaque, and gingivitis. Oil pulling is an Ayurvedic remedy that has been used to promote oral health, as well as overall well-being, for thousands of years. Repeated daily, this remedy can help whiten your teeth, freshen your breath, and more. But do not expect immediate results; it can take weeks to notice the benefits of oil pulling. Perform oil pulling first thing in the morning, preferably before you have had anything to eat or drink. **TOPICAL, SAFE FOR AGES 12+, DO NOT USE IF PREGNANT OR BREASTFEEDING, DO NOT USE WITH BLOOD THINNERS**

5 drops peppermint essential oil
3 drops clove essential oil
3 drops frankincense essential oil
3 drops myrrh essential oil
3 drops thyme essential oil
1 drop cinnamon essential oil
1 cup virgin coconut oil, barely melted

1. Put the essential oils in an 8-ounce jar and swirl to blend.
2. Pour the melted coconut oil in the jar and stir until completely blended. Cap the jar and label it. Store it in the refrigerator between uses.
3. To use, place 1 teaspoon of the blend in your mouth and allow it to melt. Swish it around and push it in and out of the spaces between your teeth for 1 to 2 minutes. Do not swallow the oil.
4. Spit the oil into the toilet or trash can. (Do not spit into the sink as the oil can cause clogging.)
5. Rinse your mouth with water, swishing between your teeth to remove excess oil. Repeat if needed, and then brush your teeth as usual. Do this daily.

TECHNIQUE TIP: Over time, increase the amount of oil you swish around your mouth to 2 to 3 teaspoons and gradually work your way up to 20-minute oil-pulling sessions (at least on occasion). When you need to spit out the oil, replace it with a fresh couple of teaspoons—the idea is to keep the same dose of oil moving through your mouth the whole time.

SELF-CARE BOOST: If you love green tea, go ahead and enjoy it often but try to skip adding sugar, which is not great for oral health. Studies show that green tea offers anti-inflammatory benefits for your gums, as well as antibacterial properties that contribute to better oral health overall.

SOOTHING PMS MASSAGE OIL

Comforting clove and balancing clary sage combine with refreshing geranium in this blend. Neroli offers antispasmodic action, helping ease physical discomfort. This soothing fragrance also eases emotional tension. If you are in a pinch and cannot create the full massage blend, clary sage can help on its own. Simply inhaling directly from the bottle or creating a simple massage with 1 drop clary sage and 1 teaspoon carrier oil can help you relax while encouraging physical and mental balance. **TOPICAL, SAFE FOR AGES 2+, DO NOT USE IF PREGNANT, DO NOT USE WITH BLOOD THINNERS**

10 drops clary sage
  essential oil
10 drops geranium
  essential oil
10 drops neroli essential oil
6 drops clove essential oil
4 ounces carrier oil

1. Put the essential oils in a 4-ounce, dark-colored bottle. Swirl to blend.

2. Add the carrier oil and cap the bottle tightly. Shake gently to mix.

3. For a soothing massage, use ¼ teaspoon of the blend to massage your neck and shoulders, stretching slowly and breathing deeply. If you suffer from serious pre-menstrual syndrome (PMS) that arrives on schedule each month, start this massage a few days before your PMS normally arrives and continue to enjoy this simple time-out for as many days as you need to.

SELF-CARE BOOST: Getting your body moving while you are experiencing PMS can be really helpful for symptoms like bloating, irritability, and fatigue, but opt for gentle exercises like walking or yoga. You know what else is really helpful for PMS symptoms? Acupuncture.

FADE MY SCARS ROLL-ON

Healing essential oils promote proper skin regeneration and can visibly reduce the appearance of scars. Anti-inflammatory frankincense and sandalwood mix with stimulating hyssop and regenerative helichrysum in this blend. You can try it on any scar, but it is best used on freshly healed wounds when scars are still forming. If you have stretch marks, this blend may help them fade as well. **TOPICAL, SAFE FOR AGES 2+, DO NOT USE IF PREGNANT OR BREASTFEEDING, DO NOT USE IF YOU HAVE EPILEPSY**

6 drops helichrysum essential oil

3 drops frankincense essential oil

3 drops sandalwood essential oil

3 drops hyssop essential oil

1¾ teaspoons jojoba oil

1. Using a fresh pipette for each oil, put the essential oils in a prelabeled 10-milliliter roller bottle. Add the jojoba oil.

2. Snap on the rollerball and screw on the cap. Shake until well-mixed.

3. Dab onto scars, using just enough to cover the area. Massage in and repeat once or twice daily during the healing process.

SELF-CARE BOOST: Honey has been used for centuries to help with wound healing and scar reduction, and several studies back this up. Try applying Manuka honey from New Zealand on your scar to speed up healing time.

SOOTHING SKIN CONDITIONER

With a base of virgin coconut oil, this blend offers antimicrobial and anti-inflammatory benefits even before you add the essential oils. Roman chamomile soothes and calms irritation, neroli clarifies and rejuvenates, and helichrysum offers anti-inflammatory, pain-relieving, and regenerative properties. Double-check that you are not allergic to any of these oils before using this treatment, even though it is very gentle. **TOPICAL, SAFE FOR AGES 2+**

20 drops neroli essential oil
10 drops helichrysum
    essential oil
10 drops Roman
    chamomile essential oil
1 cup virgin coconut oil,
    barely melted

1. Put the essential oils in an 8-ounce jar with a tight-fitting lid and swirl for about 5 seconds to blend.

2. Add the melted coconut oil and mix completely. Cap the jar, label it, and store it in a cool, dark place between uses.

3. Apply the conditioner to freshly washed skin, using as much or as little as needed to address specific areas. Start with about a pea-size amount to gauge how much you will need to use. Repeat as needed for soft, smooth skin.

SELF-CARE BOOST: Food sensitivities are a common cause of skin redness and irritation. If you notice that your skin feels "angrier" after eating common triggers like gluten or dairy, try removing them from your diet for a week or two and see if you notice a difference. Alcohol and spicy foods are common triggers, too.

COMFORTING SEA SALT GARGLE

Soothe your throat with this gargle at the first sign of irritation. Lemon, clove, and thyme contribute strong antibacterial and antiviral action to kill germs. At the same time, clove and thyme help by offering natural pain relief. During cold and flu season, you can use this gargle preemptively if you think you might have been exposed to a virus. If you are in a pinch, gargling with a dilution of even one of these essential oils will help. **TOPICAL, SAFE FOR AGES 12+, DO NOT USE IF PREGNANT OR BREASTFEEDING, DO NOT USE WITH BLOOD THINNERS**

8 ounces warm (not hot) water
½ teaspoon sea salt or Himalayan pink salt
1 drop clove essential oil
1 drop lemon essential oil
1 drop thyme essential oil

1. In a drinking glass, combine the warm water with the salt. Stir until the salt is completely dissolved. Add the essential oils to the saltwater and stir again.

2. Gargle and swish repeatedly, using 1 mouthful of the remedy at a time. Coat your throat and mouth, and then spit the liquid into the sink. Do not swallow the mixture. Wait 5 to 10 minutes before eating or drinking anything.

TECHNIQUE TIP: Although it is healing, salt can sting a severe sore throat; it is fine to omit it if it causes too much discomfort.

SELF-CARE BOOST: When you are sick, stay hydrated even though it might hurt to drink, since a dry throat is prone to further irritation. Warm liquids such as herbal tea can help. Honey is soothing and protective, too, so add a teaspoon to your tea or try honey throat drops.

SOOTHING AFTER-SUN BALM

Whether you have sustained a sunburn or you are simply looking for a way to nourish your skin after exposure to UV rays, this comforting blend can help by reducing pain, inflammation, and swelling. Together, lavender, helichrysum, and rose offer anti-inflammatory and pain-relieving properties while encouraging the skin to heal. If you like this blend, feel free to use it as one of your go-to moisturizers anytime. Your skin will thank you! **TOPICAL, SAFE FOR AGES 2+, DO NOT USE IF PREGNANT**

12 drops helichrysum essential oil

6 drops frankincense essential oil

6 drops rose essential oil

3 drops lavender essential oil

2 ounces jojoba oil

1. Put the essential oils in a 2-ounce bottle with a tight-fitting lid and swirl together for about 5 seconds.

2. Add the jojoba oil. Cap the bottle and shake well. Attach a label and store in a cool, dark place between uses.

3. Apply 2 or 3 drops of this balm to each affected area, using more or less as needed for complete coverage. Repeat 2 or 3 times daily until you recover from sunburn.

SELF-CARE BOOST: Staying hydrated is one of the easiest ways to help your skin recover from a sunburn. Pure water is best, but feel free to enjoy herbal tea and coconut water, too.

REFRESHING FOOT SPRAY

Treat your tired tootsies to a refreshing pick-me-up with this spray, which includes a combination of stimulating lemongrass, pain-relieving marjoram, energizing basil, and invigorating peppermint. If your calves and ankles are tired, feel free to give them a spritz as well. **TOPICAL, SAFE FOR AGES 6+, DO NOT USE IF PREGNANT OR BREASTFEEDING, DO NOT USE WITH DRUGS METABOLIZED BY CYP2B6**

12 drops peppermint
  essential oil
12 drops basil essential oil
6 drops marjoram
  essential oil
6 drops lemongrass
  essential oil
½ cup witch hazel

1. Put the essential oils in a bottle that can be fitted with a spray top. (If you are using a pipette to measure out the oils, use a new one for each essential oil—do not reuse.) Swirl for a few seconds to blend.

2. Add the witch hazel. Cap the bottle and shake well. Affix a label. (The witch hazel should completely emulsify the essential oils; if there is a layer of essential oil floating on top of the witch hazel, shake before each use.)

3. Pump 2 or 3 spritzes of spray onto your feet. Stretch and flex your toes and arches while the blend dries. If you can, spend a few minutes with your feet and legs comfortably propped up.

SELF-CARE BOOST: Add comfortable inserts to your shoes to provide extra cushioning, particularly if you spend a lot of time standing, walking, or running. Try not to wear anything too tight on your feet or legs since decreased circulation contributes to foot fatigue.

EMERGENCY PAIN-RELIEF BALM

If your dentist cannot see you right away, certain essential oils can temporarily relieve dental pain. Clove and cinnamon are strong pain relievers, and both offer powerful antibacterial action that can help kill bacteria that might make matters worse in the interim. This balm is not a substitute for professional dental care, so see your dentist as soon as you can. **TOPICAL, SAFE FOR AGES 12+, DO NOT USE IF PREGNANT OR BREASTFEEDING, DO NOT USE WITH BLOOD THINNERS**

15 drops cinnamon
essential oil
15 drops clove essential oil
4 tablespoons virgin
coconut oil,
barely melted

1. Put the essential oils in a 2-ounce jar with a tight-fitting lid and swirl to blend.

2. Add the coconut oil and stir until completely combined. Cap the jar and affix a label. Store the balm in the refrigerator between uses.

3. Using a clean finger, apply the balm directly onto the painful tooth, using just 1 or 2 drops at a time. If you prefer, apply the balm to a cotton ball and nestle it next to your painful tooth. Repeat as needed to numb the dental pain.

SELF-CARE BOOST: Since a dental infection can quickly travel from a tooth into your jaw and cause serious problems, it is important to get to the dentist right away when you are experiencing pain in and around your mouth. Go to the emergency room if necessary; many hospitals have dental residency programs with on-call residents who might be able to treat you in a pinch.

SOOTHING SUPPOSITORIES

This simple blend can help soothe the itch and ease the burn that often accompanies a yeast infection while killing the germs that cause it. Double-check that you are not sensitive to lavender or tea tree oil before trying this remedy. **TOPICAL, SAFE FOR AGES 16+, DO NOT USE IF PREGNANT**

6 drops tea tree essential oil
2 drops lavender essential oil
4 tablespoons virgin coconut oil, barely melted

1. In a small freezer-safe bowl that can be fitted with a lid, combine the essential oils. Add the coconut oil and stir until completely blended.

2. Place the lid on the bowl and put it in the freezer for 10 minutes. Check the blend to see if it can be molded. If not, freeze for another 10 minutes.

3. Divide the partially frozen blend into 4 equal parts. Gently mold each part into a cylindrical suppository. (These do not have to be perfectly shaped.)

4. Return the suppositories to the bowl, cover with the lid, and freeze for about 30 minutes. Store in the refrigerator or freezer between uses.

5. With clean fingers, gently insert 1 suppository into the vagina. Wear a protective pad to catch excess oil as it melts. Repeat once or twice daily for up to 2 days, preferably while you are resting overnight.

SELF-CARE BOOST: This remedy is simply intended to provide relief from vaginal itching and mild burning. Since other vaginal infections come with symptoms that are similar to those of yeast infections, it is important to be seen by your health-care practitioner, who can provide an accurate diagnosis and recommend next steps.

REFERENCES

Amsterdam, Jay D., Yimei Li, Irene Soeller, Kenneth Rockwell, Jun James Mao, and Justine Shults. "A Randomized, Double-Blind, Placebo-Controlled Trial of *Oral Matricaria recutita* (Chamomile) Extract Therapy for Generalized Anxiety Disorder." *Journal of Clinical Psychopharmacology* 29, no. 4 (August 2009): 378–82. doi. org/10.1097/JCP.0b013e3181ac935c.

Bratman, Gregory N., Gretchen C. Daily, Benjamin J. Levy, and James J. Gross. "The Benefits of Nature Experience: Improved Affect and Cognition." *Landscape and Urban Planning* 138 (June 2015): 41–50. doi.org/10.1016/j.landurbplan.2015.02.005.

Brownstein, Joe. "Planning 'Worry Time' May Help Ease Anxiety." *Live Science.* July 26, 2011. https://www.livescience.com/15233-planning-worry-time -ease-anxiety.html.

Chang, So Young. "Effects of Aroma Hand Massage on Pain, State Anxiety and Depression in Hospice Patients with Terminal Cancer." *Journal of Korean Academy of Nursing* 38, no. 4 (August 2008): 493–502. doi.org/10.4040/jkan.2008.38.4.493.

Choi, Seo Yeon, Purum Kang, Hui Su Lee, and Geun Hee Seol. "Effects of Inhalation of Essential Oil of *Citrus aurantium* L. var. *amara* on Menopausal Symptoms, Stress, and Estrogen in Postmenopausal Women: A Randomized Controlled Trial." *Evidence-Based Complementary and Alternative Medicine* 2014, no. 2 (June 2014). doi.org/10.1155/2014/796518.

Colgate-Palmolive Company. "Green Tea May Be Good for Periodontal Health: Study." The website of the Colgate-Palmolive Company. Accessed October 8, 2019. https://www.colgate.com/en-us/oral-health/conditions/gum-disease /ada-03-green-tea-may-be-good-for-periodontal-health.

Cooksley, Valerie Gennari. *Aromatherapy: A Lifetime Guide to Healing with Essential Oils.* Englewood Cliffs, NJ: Prentice Hall, 1996.

Edwards, Victoria H. *The Aromatherapy Companion: Medicinal Uses/Ayurvedic Healing/Body-Care Blends/Perfumes & Scents/Emotional Health & Well-Being.* North Adams, MA: Storey Publishing, 1999.

Gattefossé, René-Maurice. *Gattefossé's Aromatherapy: The First Book on Aroma-therapy.* Saffron Walden, UK: The C.W. Daniels Company, 1993.

Harman, Ann. *Harvest to Hydrosol: Distill Your Own Exquisite Hydrosols at Home.* Fruitland, WA: botANNicals, 2015.

HealthStatus. "Feeling Tired? Go for a Walk." The website of HealthStatus. Accessed October 8, 2019. https://www.healthstatus.com/health_blog/wellness /feeling-tired-go-for-a-walk/.

Hunter, MaryCarol Rossiter, Brenda W. Gillespie, and Sophie Yu-Pu Chen. "Urban Nature Experiences Reduce Stress in the Context of Daily Life Based on Salivary Biomarkers." *Frontiers in Psychology*, no. 10 (April 2019): 722. doi.org/10.3389 /fpsyg.2019.00722.

Jacques, Renee. "Can Your Skin-Care Routine Relieve Anxiety?" *Allure.* July 21, 2015. https://www.allure.com/story/skin-care-anxiety-relief.

Keville, Kathi and Mindy Green. *Aromatherapy: A Complete Guide to the Healing Art.* 2nd ed. New York: Crossing Press, 2009.

Kolb, Bryan, Robbin Gibb, and Terry Robinson. "Brain Plasticity and Behavior." *Current Directions in Psychological Science* 12, no. 1 (February 2003): 1–5. doi.org/10.1111/1467-8721.01210.

Lawless, Julia. *The Illustrated Encyclopedia of Essential Oils: The Complete Guide to the Use of Oils in Aromatherapy and Herbalism.* Rockport, MA: Element Books, 1995.

Lis-Balchin, Maria. *Aromatherapy Science: A Guide for Healthcare Professionals.* Grayslake, IL: Pharmaceutical Press, 2006.

LoBisco, Sarah. "Essential Oils for Mood Support." Saratoga.com. May 8, 2018. https://www.saratoga.com/healing-health-wellness/2018/05 /essential-oils-for-mood-support/.

Manniche, Lise. *Sacred Luxuries: Fragrance, Aromatherapy, and Cosmetics in Ancient Egypt.* Ithaca, NY: Cornell University Press, 1999.

Molan, P. C. "The Evidence Supporting the Use of Honey as a Wound Dressing." *The International Journal of Lower Extremity Wounds* 5, no. 1 (March 2006): 40–54. doi. org/10.1177/1534734605286014.

Moss, Mark and Lorraine Oliver. "Plasma 1,8-Cineole Correlates with Cognitive Performance Following Exposure to Rosemary Essential Oil Aroma." *Therapeutic Advances in Psychopharmacology* 2, no. 3 (June 2012): 103–13. doi .org/10.1177/2045125312436573.

Price, Shirley. *Aromatherapy Workbook: A Complete Guide to Understanding and Using Essential Oils.* London: Thorsons, 1993.

Saito, Naoko, Emi Yamano, Akira Ishii, Masaaki Tanaka, Junji Nakamura, and Yasuyoshi Watanabe. "Involvement of the Olfactory System in the Induction of Anti-Fatigue Effects by Odorants." *PLOS ONE* 13, no. 3 (March 2018). doi.org/10.1371/journal .pone.0195263.

Saiyudthong, Somrudee, and Charles A. Marsden. "Acute Effects of Bergamot Oil on Anxiety-Related Behaviour and Corticosterone Level in Rats." *Phytotherapy Research* 25, no. 6 (June 2011): 858–62. doi.org/10.1002/ptr.3325.

Schnaubelt, Kurt. *Medical Aromatherapy: Healing with Essential Oils.* Berkeley: Frog Books, 1999.

Tisserand, Robert B. *The Art of Aromatherapy: The Healing and Beautifying Properties of the Essential Oils of Flowers and Herbs.* Rochester, VT: Healing Arts Press, 1977.

Tisserand, Robert B., and Rodney Young. *Essential Oil Safety: A Guide for Health Care Professionals.* 2nd ed. London: Churchill Livingstone, 2014.

Tober, Carsten, and Roland Schoop. "Modulation of Neurological Pathways by *Salvia officinalis* and Its Dependence on Manufacturing Process and Plant Parts Used." *BMC Complementary and Alternative Medicine* 19, no. 1 (December 2019): 128. doi. org/10.1186/s12906-019-2549-x.

Vecchio, Laura M., Ying Meng, Kristiana Xhima, Nir Lipsman, Clement Hamani, and Isa-belle Aubert. "The Neuroprotective Effects of Exercise: Maintaining a Healthy Brain Throughout Aging." *Brain Plasticity* 4, no. 1 (December 2018): 17–52. doi .org/10.3233/BPL-180069.

Webb, Marion. "Increase Energy Levels and Cure Fatigue Through Exercise." The website of the American Council on Exercise. September 8, 2011. https://www

.acefitness.org/education-and-resources/lifestyle/blog/6589/increase-energy-levels-and-cure-fatigue-through-exercise.

White, Gregory Lee. *Essential Oils and Aromatherapy: How to Use Essential Oils for Beauty, Health, and Spirituality. N.p.*: White Willow Books, 2013. Kindle.

Woodside, Courtney. "STUDY: 'Sugar Rush' Isn't Real, but 'Sugar Crash' Is." The website of the PAC 98.7 radio station. April 8, 2019. https://pac987fm .com/2019/04/08/study-sugar-rush-isnt-real-but-sugar-crash-is/.

Worwood, Valerie Ann. *The Complete Book of Essential Oils and Aromatherapy: Over 800 Natural, Nontoxic, and Fragrant Recipes to Create Health, Beauty, and Safe Home and Work Environments*. Novato, CA: New World Library, 1991.

Worwood, Valerie Ann. *The Fragrant Mind: Aromatherapy for Personality, Mind, Mood, and Emotion*. Novato, CA: New World Library, 1996.

Zabirunnisa, Md., Jayaprakash S. Gadagi, Praveen Gadde, Nagamalleshwari Myla, Jyothirmai Koneru, and Chandrasekhar Thatimatla. "Dental Patient Anxiety: Possible Deal with *Lavender* Fragrance." *Journal of Research in Pharmacy Practice* 3, no. 3 (July 2014): 100–03. doi.org/10.4103/2279-042X.141116.

RESOURCES

APPS

Calm: www.calm.com (Calm for Apple devices and Calm–Meditate, Sleep, Relax for Android)

Headspace: Meditation for Sleep: www.headspace.com (for Apple and Android devices)

BOOKS

Bernstein, Gabrielle. *The Universe Has Your Back: Transform Fear to Faith.* Carlsbad, CA: Hay House, 2016.

Chopra, Deepak. *The Seven Spiritual Laws of Success: A Practical Guide to the Fulfillment of Your Dreams.* San Rafael, CA: Amber-Allen, 1994.

Lipman, Frank. *How to Be Well: The 6 Keys to a Happy and Healthy Life.* New York: Houghton Mifflin Harcourt, 2018.

Raupp, Aimee E. *Body Belief: How to Heal Autoimmune Diseases, Radically Shift Your Health, and Learn to Love Your Body More.* 2nd ed. Carlsbad, CA: Hay House, 2019.

Rubin, Gretchen. *The Happiness Project: Or, Why I Spent a Year Trying to Sing in the Morning, Clean My Closets, Fight Right, Read Aristotle, and Generally Have More Fun.* New York: HarperCollins, 2011.

Sincero, Jen. *You Are a Badass: How to Stop Doubting Your Greatness and Start Living an Awesome Life.* Philadelphia: Running Press, 2013.

Tisserand, Robert, and Rodney Young. *Essential Oil Safety: A Guide for Health Care Professionals.* 2nd ed. London: Churchill Livingstone, 2014.

VIDEOS

TED (TED Talk video playlist). "The Importance of Self-Care." Accessed October 8, 2019. www.ted.com/playlists/299/the_importance_of_self_care.

WEBSITES

National Association for Holistic Aromatherapy: www.naha.org/education/approved-schools
List of approved schools for aromatherapy continuing education.

Tisserand Institute: www.tisserandinstitute.org/essential-oil-dilution-chart
Downloadable essential-oil dilution chart.

INDEX

ACKNOWLEDGMENTS

To Callisto Media and especially to my editor Rachel Feldman:
Thank you for inviting me on this journey!

To Anne Kennedy:
Thank you for all the hard work and research you put into this product. I learned so much and am so grateful for your knowledge.

To Randie:
Thanks for dreaming this dream for me. I remember laughing when you told me I would write a book someday. I guess you really meant multiple books!

To my little bubbies, Sadie and Remy:
You make me so proud and I love being your mama bear.

To my family:
Thank you for your love and support.

To my incredible network of friends, old and new:
Thank you for your support and encouragement.

To my colleagues, especially Elissa Ranney, Nancy Byrne, and Kelly Liberty:
Thank you for being part of my dream. I cannot wait to see what comes next!

To my patients at Indigo Acupuncture + Wellness:
Thank you for letting me share in your lives and your stories and for trusting me with your care. I am so grateful for you and honored to work with you.

ABOUT THE AUTHOR

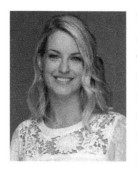 **SARAH SWANBERG, MS, LAC,** is a licensed acupuncturist and board-certified Diplomate in Oriental Medicine through the National Certification Commission for Acupuncture and Oriental Medicine (NCCAOM). She holds a master of science in Traditional Oriental Medicine from the Pacific College of Oriental Medicine (PCOM) in New York City. In her practice, Indigo Acupuncture + Wellness, located in Stamford, Connecticut, Sarah combines the time-honored art of Chinese medicine with practical health advice for the modern world. She lives in Stamford, Connecticut, with her husband and two daughters. You can find her at IndigoAcu. com or on Instagram at @IndigoAcu.

CPSIA information can be obtained
at www.ICGtesting.com
Printed in the USA
JSHW011130100620
6152JS00001B/1